THE
STRESS
FACTOR

Previously published in Britain under the title
Executive Stress: Strategies for Survival

Donald Norfolk

SIMON AND SCHUSTER · New York

PUBLISHED BY SIMON & SCHUSTER
A DIVISION OF GULF & WESTERN CORPORATION
SIMON & SCHUSTER BUILDING
ROCKEFELLER CENTER
1230 AVENUE OF THE AMERICAS
NEW YORK, NEW YORK 10020
DESIGNED BY DIANNE PINKOWITZ
MANUFACTURED IN THE UNITED STATES OF AMERICA
1 2 3 4 5 6 7 8 9 10

LIBRARY OF CONGRESS CATALOGING IN PUBLICATION DATA

Norfolk, Donald, date.
    The stress factor.

    Bibliography: p.
    Includes index.
    1. Stress (Psychology)   2. Stress (Phys-
iology)   3. Work—Psychological aspects.
    I. Title.
    BF575.S75N67   158'.1   78-13484

    ISBN 0-671-24275-X

CONTENTS

PART III   THE CONTROL OF STRESS

Part I
THE BIOLOGY OF STRESS

1
THE STRESS OF LIFE

Stress, like hunger and thirst, is an inescapable part of life. We experience it when we drive a car through busy traffic, burn a finger on the stove, have a nightmare, fight with the children, or try to fill out a complicated tax return. Attempts to define it invariably fail. A search of the medical literature shows that there are over three hundred different definitions of anxiety, and none of these can be considered wholly satisfactory.

Although stress is an integral part of our everyday lives, it remains remarkably little understood. A few years ago a group of research workers and doctors carried out an eighteen-month study of stress in industry, which revealed "a dearth of facts, and a plethora of unproved assumptions." Numerous papers have been published on the subject, but most have been written in technical language for the specialist reader—doctor, industrial psychologist, biochemist and social scientist. This book draws heavily on these sources but is written in terms that the intelligent laymen can easily understand. It is intended as a practical guide and includes advice received during interviews with a large number of people from many different walks of life, including actors, film producers, storekeepers, business administrators, government officials, school principals, accountants, architects and company directors. Throughout the book the subject under stress is generally referred to for convenience as *he*, although it is realized that it could just as easily be *she*. In fact many of the female subjects interviewed pointed out that women at work frequently suffer more stress than their male co-workers because they have to combine their jobs with running a home, caring for their husbands and coping with the children's ailments. There is no one to prepare a meal for them when they come home exhausted from the office in the evening, or to wash, iron and darn their clothes.

The book explains in Part Two the origins of stress and in Part Three suggests a variety of ways in which stress can be harnessed, handled and controlled.

When stress is handled effectively it provides the motivation which encourages us to overcome the obstacles that separate us from our hopes and goals. When it is allowed to get out of control it leads to sickness, low-level performance and premature death. It is a vital early warning system which makes us aware of situations that threaten our happiness, health, safety, self-esteem and mental equilibrium.

Some people have a high tolerance for stress. This is a characteristic of successful managers. According to a study carried out by *Fortune* magazine, the quality that most clearly differentiates successful top executives from those who remain at the bottom of the ladder is "stability under pressure." Financier J. Paul Getty suggested that when candidates for an executive position appear to be of equal stature, the important question to be asked is "Which of the two men reacted best under stress?" This has always been the hallmark of the successful leader. As Beowulf the Dane says in Europe's oldest epic poem in a nonclassical language, "Fortune is apt to favor the man who keeps his nerve." One purpose of this book is to describe the ways in which this valuable quality can be acquired. It is possible to *learn* to remain calm when under pressure. Some people may be born placid, but others have to achieve the gift by careful self-training. Ideally, instruction in techniques for coping with stress should form an integral part of every comprehensive management training program. But this book is less interested in what industry, governments or institutions should do to lessen the impact of psychological strain. It is written primarily to show you, the individual reader, what *you* can do to enjoy the stimulus of stress without suffering any of its unfortunate aftereffects.

During the coming years your health, happiness and success will depend to a very large extent on your ability to adapt successfully to the stresses you meet. Failure to adapt will mean sickness, depression, loss of self-esteem and low achievement.

Many people today are aware that they are suffering from excessive stress. A study of a large group of Swedish government officials revealed that while all but two percent liked their work, eighty-two percent of them found it either occasionally or constantly stressful. Research has also revealed the high incidence of stress disorders among airline pilots. One British airline has reported that nearly fifty percent of its medical groundings were due to psychiatric disease. Even the nation's politicians are not immune.

An inquiry, conducted by the British Heart Foundation, showed that British politicians are generally physically fit but "have a high incidence of minor stress symptoms," their commonest complaints being fatigue (forty-four percent), irritability (thirty-nine percent), indigestion (thirty percent), headaches (twenty-nine percent), depression (twenty-one percent) and insomnia (twenty-three percent).

Most people have at least a vague idea of the sources of anxiety and tension in their lives. Airline pilots frequently blame the strain of shift work, jet lag and frequent absences from home. Politicians refer to long sessions, narrow government majorities and feelings of frustration and futility. A social worker in an interview with a Sunday newspaper blamed "the frustration of not being able to do one single thing properly because of the multiplicity of demands; the lack of necessary resources and facilities to do the right thing even when you have decided what should be done; the insoluble problems where there is simply no answer; and the overwhelming feeling that if anything at all goes wrong, it will all come back on me."

The Swedish bureaucrats when questioned spoke of the weight of responsibility placed upon them, lack of time, "too much to do," the need for constant attentiveness, and the confusion caused by unclear instructions and lack of information. Similar factors recur in other reports. Robert Kahn, a psychologist working at the University of Michigan's Institute for Social Research, carried out a survey throughout the United States and found widespread evidence of industrial stress. Of the employees he questioned, forty-eight percent complained of conflicting work demands, forty-five percent of work overload and thirty-five percent of lack of clarity in the scope and responsibilities of their work. Other commonly reported problems were difficult bosses and subordinates, lack of adequate participation in the decision-making process and worry over being responsible for other people. Once these sources of stress have been identified, it is normally possible to develop strategies to regulate them or keep them under effective control. This is discussed in detail in Chapters 4 to 14.

Only when stress is allowed to become excessive does it give rise to strain and sickness. Most people can provide a list of "stress" disorders such as peptic ulcers, hypertension and coronary disease; the link between these ailments and environmental distress is now fairly well established. For example, when Dr. Edward Weiss and his colleagues at the Temple University Hospital, Philadelphia, studied a group of coronary patients, they found that their heart attacks had been preceded by "gradually mounting tension" in forty-nine percent of the cases studied, and by "acute emotional stress" in thirty-seven percent. When they compared the histories of an equal number of non-coronary patients they found that none had been admitted to the hospital after a period of "gradually mounting stress" and only nine percent after an episode of sudden emotional strain. But it is wrong to associate these ailments with the successful managerial classes, for in fact both coronary disease and duodenal ulcers are more common among unskilled workers than among the managerial and professional classes. An inquiry carried out by the British Institute of Management showed that there was "no discernible occupational hazard connected with the job of being an executive." They found that executives on the average live longer than the wage earners they supervise and longer than the professional classes. Unfortunately, even doctors help to promote the myth that these are primarily the "boss's" diseases. When Professor Laurence Peter asked a number of doctors what diseases they associated with "success" they provided him with a formidable array of psychosomatic ailments. The list included peptic ulcers, colitis, high blood pressure, constipation, alcoholism, fibrositis, insomnia, chronic fatigue, migraine, heart disease, dizziness, impotence and nervous dermatitis. But, as Professor Peter pointed out in his wise and witty book *The Peter Principle*, the widespread occurrence of these ailments among managers is merely a sad indication that many of them have been promoted to a level at which they are incapable of coping with the stresses placed upon them. In positions of responsibility our health and efficiency depend on how well we cope with our environment, and the evidence is that the successful executive positively thrives in a milieu of turmoil and strife. As the novelist Arnold Bennett wrote in *Mental Efficiency*, "The average man flourishes in an atmosphere of peaceful routine. Men destined for success flourish and find their ease in an atmosphere of collision and disturbance."

A survey taken at the Bell Telephone Company showed that switchboard workers have twice as many heart attacks as the company's top executives. This is confirmed by actuarial studies which show that the death rate among company presidents is only fifty-eight percent of the average for the country's white males. It seems that contrary to popular belief, stress, far from hastening a successful manager to an early demise, actually helps to prolong his life. This is particularly noticeable among American Presidents, many of whom have lived to a venerable age. It has been shown that U.S. Presidents, unless they meet an unnatural death, live longer on average than Vice-Presidents, and longer still than unsuccessful candidates for the Presidency. Experiments conducted by Professor W. S. Bullough, Professor of Zoology at Birkbeck College, London, show that mice, whose normal life span is two years, can be made to live twice as long if they are subjected to repeated stress. This is probably because exposure to intermittent stress stimulates the adrenal glands and keeps the body's defense mechanisms working at peak efficiency.

A regular shot of adrenaline is also a wonderful cure for lethargy and boredom. This again has been confirmed by experiments on laboratory animals. The National Institute of Mental Health built a veritable paradise for mice stocked with every conceivable comfort and food. But ennui rapidly occurred in this rodent Garden of Eden. The youngsters became listless, the mice of reproductive age lost their sexual urge and the older members of the population showed increasing signs of stress. The entire community lost their interest and zest for life and their ability to recognize and respond to challenge. Psychiatrists report that while depression has become increasingly common in Britain, it has shown a marked decrease in areas of Northern Ireland most heavily affected by outbreaks of violence and civil disturbance. No doubt the continual presence of danger has stimulated people's output of stress hormones, which act as powerful pep pills. That also explains why many people leading drab, uneventful lives go out of their way to enjoy the stimulus of risk-taking activities like rock climbing, caving and car racing. And why so many business tycoons seek out the excitement of the gambling tables the moment they are financially secure. We need the stimulus of occasional anxiety and fear to keep us alert and alive.

The time to worry is when you stop worrying. Stress prods us into action. If this action is blocked by some external agency we become frustrated, and this makes us redouble our efforts to secure our goal. Anxiety is also beneficial, for it increases our level of arousal and helps us perform at peak efficiency. As the world-famous photographer Karsh of Ottawa avers, we generally give of our best when we're under stress. "I judge the success of a sitting by the number of hours of sleep I lost the night before," he says.

Psychologists have repeatedly proved the soundness of the Yerkes-Dodson law. This is probably the only example of a truly scientific psychological law. It states that anxiety improves performance until a certain optimum level of arousal has been reached. Beyond that point performance deteriorates as higher levels of anxiety are attained. In practice, the important thing is to recognize when we have achieved an optimum level and then refuse to be pressured beyond this point. As Professor Hans Selye, the world's greatest authority on stress, said. "The goal is certainly not to avoid stress . . . there is no more justification for avoiding stress than for shunning food, exercise or love. But in order to express yourself fully you must first find your optimum stress level."

The chapter which follows offers some practical advice on how to recognize your own level of optimum stress arousal. Faced with this knowledge it is possible to enjoy the excitement, *élan vital* and creative driving force which stress affords without suffering any of its harmful consequences. This is the ability above all else that separates the leaders of industry from their subordinates. The timid run away from challenging situations; the bold accept the opportunities they provide for development and growth.

The Chinese use two pictures to depict the concept of "crisis." They link the symbol for danger with the symbol for opportunity, thus expressing their belief that every crisis provides an opportunity. Those who learn to cope with stress have the confidence and ability to seize the opportunities of life without suffering its hurts.

2
THE WORRYING KIND

Many executives are notoriously unwilling to admit that they are under stress. They love to be in the thick of the fray, and when tensions and frustrations mount they merely redouble their efforts and extend the pace and length of their working day. These are the world's workaholics who, unless they are careful, will continue to push themselves a little harder until the break finally comes and they succumb to a heart attack or nervous breakdown. Then they invariably express surprise. "I never thought this would happen to me," they say. "I'm not the worrying kind. I've always been able to cope with any amount of stress without showing the slightest sign of strain."

Others magnify the pressures they are under. While the office cleaner moans about her rheumatism, they constanly gripe about the stress and strain of modern life, their impossible work load, exhausting traveling schedules and heavy burden of responsibility. They couldn't survive without the support of tranquilizers, sleeping pills, whiskey and strong black coffee. And even with the aid of these pick-me-ups, they are convinced that, sooner or later, they are going to join the company's steadily mounting casualty list. Maybe their grumbling peptic ulcer will finally break down and hemorrhage, or perhaps they will have a coronary or a prolonged bout of depression like so many of their colleagues.

These tales of woe frequently include two fallacies. The first is the belief that there exists a race of executive supermen who are totally immune to stress. The second is the myth of "the increased stress of modern life." Both these ideas are false. Crossing the Atlantic Ocean in a pressurized jet can hardly be more stressful than rolling and pitching for weeks on end in an overloaded schooner. And traveling from New York to Washington, D.C., in an air-conditioned, high-speed train can hardly produce as much nervous strain as our forbears experienced driving over potholed roads in a stagecoach which could at any time be robbed. Each age provides its own particular stress and strain. The problem is that we have not yet learned to cope with ours. This is because life has changed more rapidly than our powers of adaptation. In many ways life today is far *less* stressful than it was before. There is no need for us to break down under its weight and suffer insomnia, headaches, hypertension, ulcers, fatigue and depression. But with the rapid change in our lifestyle, we can no longer sit back and rely on the automatic protection provided by psychological coping techniques which take generations to evolve. In a world that is in a state of constant flux, each generation must consciously develop its own survival strategies. If we are to thrive as individuals we must take stock and see how stress affects our lives, how it can be harnessed to maximum advantage, and how its excesses can be avoided. The whole purpose of this book is to facilitate this process.

It is a task that nobody should shirk. No one is in so lowly a position that he can escape the impact of stress, and no one is so invulnerable that he is totally immune from its effect. Experience during two world wars has shown that even the hardiest soldiers will break down and suffer "shell shock" or battle fatigue if they are subjected to sufficient strain. The same applies to political prisoners. Modern brainwashing techniques will bring even the toughest, most stoical subjects to the point of nervous collapse if they are forced to endure the stress of too much noise, bright lights, insufficient sleep and physical deprivation.

Some people, however, can withstand more stress than others. Just as we vary in height, strength, intelligence and color of hair, so we differ in our tolerance to stress. Hippocrates, the father of modern medicine, believed that people could be classified into four basic personality types —the choleric, the sanguine, the phlegmatic and the melancholic. He noted that our reaction to life's problems depends not only on the situation itself, but also on our underlying temperament. This accords well with the observations made almost two thousand years later by Ivan Pavlov, the great Russian physiologist. He showed that it is possible to bring about a rupture of nervous activity in any animal if it is subjected to a sufficient level of stress. In some animals this is considerably easier than in others. After studying the physiological response of dogs for thirty years he found that it was possible to divide the animals into four categories according to their reaction to stress. His grouping proved to be practically identical to that of Hippocrates. He described a "strong excitatory" type (choleric); a "lively" type (sanguine); a "calm imperturbable" type (phlegmatic) and a "weak inhibitory" type (melancholic). It was found that the "strong excitatory" animals became wild and out of control when faced with conflict or stress; the "lively" ones became excited, but their behavior remained more purposeful and controlled; the "calm imperturbable" ones showed a more passive reaction, while the "weak inhibitory" animals rapidly showed a form of fear paralysis. Similar reactions to frustrations can be seen in humans.

William Sargant, Honorary Consultant Psychiatrist at St. Thomas's Hospital, London, has made a detailed study of human behavior under stress, both in times of war and when undergoing scientifically applied brainwashing procedures. He reports: "Persons of phlegmatic temperament and strong heavy body-build, who are also mentally well adjusted with a settled, happy viewpoint on life, are likely to hold out longer than those who have few or none of these assets." Pavlov believed that although these basic temperaments are inherited, they are also open to environmental modification.

Ideally, we should adopt job selection procedures which ensure that the more demanding occupations are offered only to people with a high level of stress tolerance. This would undoubtedly reduce the level of psychosomatic illness in industry, as it has done in the army, where the introduction of a more careful psychological screening of recruits has reduced the psychiatric casualty rate from ten percent in the Second World War to one percent during the war in Vietnam. In addition, the scope of management training should be extended to include the understanding and management of stress. The competent manager must increase his tolerance for stress so that he can welcome rather than shirk the challenges of life. He must develop the ability to remain unflustered in a crisis and in a position to support his co-workers and subordinates by his mien of quiet confidence and easy composure. Even if we are by nature a choleric type, likely to fly off the handle at the slightest provocation, we can learn to control our emotional outbursts. If we are inherently melancholic we can, by patient training, develop the knack of reacting positively rather than negatively to life's rebuffs.

This, however, demands a far higher degree of self-understanding than most people possess. Many ambitious businessmen will go to great lengths to understand the intricacies of computer technology, corporate law and capital investment theories, yet fail to study their most valuable managerial tool—themselves. This is not difficult to understand. Our behavior is often so irrational, so immature, so idiosyncratic that we would not want to examine it too closely. Frequently we recapitulate behavior patterns that were established and found to be effective in childhood, but which are wholly inappropriate to our current situation. If we found we could get our own way in the nursery by throwing a temper tantrum, we may still try to do the same thing in the boardroom, but with totally different results. Acknowledgment of this immature behavior may be painful, but the more we recognize these atavistic behavioral quirks, the greater the chance that we can control our emotional outbursts and irrational behavior and achieve maturity.

Techniques for achieving this level of understanding include:

- *Analyze your strengths and weaknesses.* According to J. Paul Getty, "The business executive must be able to appraise his own capabilities and limitations honestly. He should form the habit of periodically making an objective inventory of himself, doing it, if necessary, literally, using pencil and paper." How much competition can you take? Do you need the security of a large corporation? Are you good at handling people?

Everyone has talents, but no man can do everything supremely well. The ideal is to exploit your strengths and protect your weaknesses. But this can only be done when we genuinely acknowledge our deficiencies. Stress arises when we are constantly struggling to conceal our limitations and maintain a pose of inauthentic competency.

One of the most misused phrases in the psychologists' lexicon is "inferiority complex." We do not become neurotic simply because we are a dwarf, impotent or dyslexic. We develop a neurosis when we try to deny and overcompensate for these deficiencies. Life is much easier when we offer ourselves as we are. As Matthew Arnold advised: "Resolve to be thyself; and know that he who finds himself, loses his misery." We are also likely to achieve a greater measure of success when we are not wasting time and effort in constant playacting. Dr. Robert Murray, a consultant psychologist, studied a large group of men who failed to make a success of their jobs even though they were well trained, physically fit and above average in intelligence. He found that the major reason for their failure was that they were unable to acknowledge any kind of personal limitation. Theirs was what Thomas Carlyle described as the greatest of all faults—to be conscious of none.

Weaknesses should be acknowledged and strengths relentlessly exploited. Macbeth was a brilliant military commander but an incompetent king.

Hitler was a powerful, effective politician but an incompetent military commander. Socrates was a consummate teacher, but an ineffectual defense lawyer. Excitement may come from embarking on a totally fresh task. Contentment comes from undertaking what we know we can do well, and doing it a little better.

- *Clarify your goals.* (This will be discussed in greater detail in Chapter 5.) Many managers show an amazing degree of uncertainty and ambivalence about their aspirations and goals. Few have analyzed the extent of their ambitions, their need for status and power, the significance to them of salary levels, or the relative importance of family, friends, pastimes and job. Others suffer stress because they struggle through life with conflicting goals. Frequently the ethical standards they uphold in private life differ from those they maintain at work. This means an inevitable loss of self-esteem, and tests show that high levels of anxiety are often associated with a low level of self-esteem. Nothing succeeds like success; but to succeed we must know the goals at which we are aiming. This calls for some soul-searching self-examination. We need to find the answer to such fundamental questions as: What is the purpose of my life? What are the ethical standards I want to maintain? What are the values I want to pass on to my children? What are the goals I hope to achieve?

  There is bound to be a discrepancy between the person we are and the person we would like to be. But the narrower the gap the less stress we suffer and the greater contentment we feel. We must, above all else, endeavor to be at peace with ourselves. And this requires a definite philosophy of life, a code of ethics and a set of clearly stated aims.

- *Study what causes you stress.* No two people react to stress in quite the same way. One person may revel in frequent change, while another may be thrown into a state of considerable disquiet if his telephone is moved to the opposite side of the desk. A manager may come unscathed through a long takeover battle, or travel on a whirlwind, round-the-world trip in search of new business, and yet quake at the thought of rising to his feet to give an after-dinner speech at his daughter's wedding. Once we establish the origins of stress in our individual lives, we can set about the task of modifying its impact. This is dealt with in detail in the second section of this book. Locating the source of our anxieties has of itself a therapeutic effect. As Dr. Hans Selye said, "The mere fact of knowing what hurts has a curative value."

- *Recognize the symptoms of stress.* No alarm bells ring to show when we are suffering undue stress, but there are adequate warning signs. People under stress generally become more irritable and over-react to relatively trivial frustrations. They show a change in their sleep pattern, they step up their drinking and smoking and become increasingly tired and restless. They derive fewer pleasures from life. They laugh less and become plagued with feelings of inadequacy and self-doubt, which makes them constantly check their own and other people's work. As the strain mounts, their memory fails and their powers of concentration wane. They also develop psychosomatic ailments such as tension headaches, indigestion and colitis. Most people tend to have their own target organs, which are the first to suffer when they are under stress. Harold Wilson suffered stomach pains whenever he had to fire a colleague. Henry Ford, whenever he had to make an important business decision, developed stomach cramps which were sometimes so severe that he was left writhing on the floor. When Mussolini was working under pressure he had to take frequent sips of milk to calm his nagging peptic ulcer, and in these circumstances Trotsky developed bouts of high temperature which frequently forced him to retire to the Crimea to recuperate.

Once we recognize our own particular pattern of stress symptomatology we can take steps to introduce early prophylactic treatment along the lines described in the third section of this book.

• *Understand your favored coping techniques.* The way we react to stress depends on the basic defense mechanisms we acquired in childhood to cope with anxiety. Freud described nine basic psychological defense mechanisms. Several others have since been added to the list, bringing the number up to about two dozen. The most important of these psychological defense strategies are avoidance, denial, repression, projection, regression and obsessive behavior. Each of these mechanisms is employed in everyday life, and to a certain extent our personalities are shaped by the defenses we habitually use. If we find it difficult to make up our minds we may protect ourselves by following a policy of avoidance, shunning every situation in which we may be required to make a snap decision. If the company we own and run is going bankrupt we may decide to shield ourselves by denying that things are as black as they seem. We may use the technique of repression to bury in our subconscious mind any feelings of inadequacy or insecurity. We can, if we choose, disown our aggressive tendencies and attribute them to belligerent co-workers, just as a spinster may project her sexual feelings onto the sinful world around her. If the pressures of life get too severe we may slip into a position of increased dependency on the state, drugs, religion, business colleagues or friends; or we may derive solace by performing comforting rituals, much as a nervous child obtains reassurance by executing a set ritual before retiring to bed. These are some of the ways in which the healthy mind protects itself. Harm is done only when these responses are excessive or inappropriate.

A manager who tackles his fear of flying by a policy of strict avoidance greatly limits his usefulness if he steadfastly refuses to set foot in a plane. The executive who copes with anxiety by slipping into obsessive rituals of desk tidying and pencil straightening wastes both time and nervous energy. If our major defense mechanism is repression, and we use it excessively, we run the risk of becoming inhibited and withdrawn. If projection is our favorite protective strategy and we give it too free a rein, we run the risk of becoming critical, intolerant and hostile. If we overuse regression, we become uncomfortably dependent, demanding and irresponsible; if we exaggerate the protective use of obsessive rituals, we become narrow and rigid, and if we walk about in blinkers constantly denying the obvious, we tend to become stubborn and unimaginative.

The ideal is to develop a wide range of coping techniques and to use them as the occasion demands. That is the sign of true maturity. We cannot fail to generate emotional tension if we try to solve adult problems in a childish fashion. Tests show that there is no direct relationship between intelligence and coping ability. We handle stress successfully only if we have mastered the basic techniques of psychological survival and have the imagination and flexibility to use them appropriately. That is the mark of the true leader who, even in a crisis, will remain "sober, steady and calm." These qualities may be partly inherited, but they can also be painstakingly acquired, as subsequent chapters of this book relate.

3

THE SURVIVAL OF
THE FITTEST

A battle is waged whenever we are under stress, or our bodies are invaded by pathogenic bacteria. The outcome of these battles depends partly on the power and virulence of the assault, and partly on the effectiveness of our defenses. If a man whose defenses are weakened by malnutrition comes into contact with a few isolated pathogens he can easily develop pneumonia and die. When he is fit his body has little difficulty in destroying a handful of invading germs. The same applies when we are under stress.

The body shows a resistance to hostile attacks which is partly general and partly specific. When we inhale samples of the tubercle bacillus in a crowded bus or subway, our ability to destroy the germs and escape a full-blown attack of tuberculosis depends on our general health, and also on our specific immunity to the *mycobacterium tuberculosis*. In the same way we may face the emotional stress of sudden bereavement by employing the specific psychological defense techniques of dependency or denial, but our ability to cope with this crisis also depends on our general level of well-being. Whatever the stress we are under, we are far more likely to show signs of mental breakdown if at the time we are physically below par, anemic, or suffering from lack of sleep.

Dr. Hans Selye became a firm advocate of physical fitness as a result of a series of experiments he carried out in his Montreal laboratory. He took ten under-exercised laboratory rats and subjected them repeatedly to a variety of stresses—shocks, pain, shrill noises and blinding flashing lights. At the end of a month every one of these rats had died from the incessant strain. Then he took another sample of rats accurately matched for age and breed. These he trained with exercises on a treadmill until they were in the peak of physical condition. He then subjected them to the same battery of stresses and found they showed remarkably greater tolerance than their unfit siblings. At the end of a month none of the healthy rats had died, convincing evidence that physically fit animals can withstand stress far more easily than those who are out of condition.

Many businessmen suffer sickness and premature death simply because they have failed to apply their intelligence and business acumen to the task of keeping themselves fit. Joseph Collier, the English draper who built the multimillion United Drapery Stores Group from an initial capital stake of only £30, is typical of the many men who in their fight to get to the top fail to protect their most vital asset—their personal health. He had to retire early because of failing health, and shortly before he died from a heart attack he said: "In this drive of mine to expand, I'm afraid I neglected my health. It's the only thing I still want and I can't have it."

In Great Britain, it is estimated that one in three company directors will not live long enough to collect their pensions. They spend their lives battling for their companies but fail to preserve their own health. As a result they succumb to stress diseases, which are more easily palliated than cured. The manager who suffers a heart attack may keep going with the help of beta-blocking drugs and a slightly curtailed work program, but this is no substitute for a clean bill of health and a life untrammeled by physical restraints. Performing gastrectomies to treat a chronic ulcer is not a "cure," any more than decapitation is a panacea for recurrent headaches. Health is never acquired by treating disease. Vitality, stamina, *joie de vivre* and a high tolerance to stress are the result and direct rewards of achieving a high level of physical fitness. This is nature's way of seeing that only the fittest flourish and survive.

Many executives now realize this and are making more serious efforts to improve their health. Some organizations also encourage their key employees to keep themselves fit. Volvo, Sweden's largest motor manufacturer, insists that every executive must exercise strenuously for thirty minutes every week, either in the firm's gymnasium or over a specially designed cross-country course. The Rockwell Corporation permits its employees to have time off work three times a week to keep themselves trim. This is a sensible policy, for as Dr. Richard Morrison, the company's physical fitness expert, says: "A healthier executive is a more efficient employee."

There are five main reasons why exercise helps us cope with stress:

- *It reduces our level of anxiety.* It is possible to produce a state of extreme anxiety by injecting a solution of lactic acid into the bloodstream of ex-

perimental subjects. Less marked rises occur naturally when we are under stress or suffering from
extreme fatigue. When we exercise and breathe
more deeply we increase our intake of oxygen and
so speed up the rate at which the lactic acid is oxi-
dized and removed from the circulation. Experiments with students also demonstrate the sedative
effect of exercise during periods of stress. Psychologist Richard Driscoll of Tennessee took a group
of students suffering from pre-examination nerves
and subjected them to a variety of treatments. Afterward an assessment was made of their level of anxiety both before and after their exams. It was found
that anxiety could be reduced by a process of de-
sensitization, a technique in which the students
listened to tapes which taught them how to relax
while they faced up to their specific problems and
fears. More marked improvement was made by a
group of students whose treatment consisted of jogging while thinking about pleasant, relaxing situations. This group showed the greatest decrease in
their anxiety and the maximum improvement in
their examination marks. As Richard Driscoll concluded in an article in *The Psychological Review,*
jogging is a simpler, quicker way of reducing anxiety than the far more elaborate technique of de-
sensitization. It can be practiced anywhere, needs
no therapist and requires only the barest minimum
of equipment.

- *It provides a socially acceptable form of abreaction.*
  Every animal has its own way of letting off steam.
  Antelopes, instead of fighting with a rival, may
  clash their antlers against a tree. Birds will tear up

grass. When we are frustrated, we will stamp our feet, swear, throw books, slam doors or kick the cat. A more civilized form of catharsis is to play a game of tennis or jog around the park.

- *It builds up stamina.* The executive who is fit is in a far better position to cope with prolonged and complicated working schedules. Julius Caesar may have asked to have around him men who were fat, but he would have been much better served by acolytes who were athletic and slim. Such men perform better themselves and are also more likely to enthuse their followers. As Carl Duerr says in *Management Kinetics*: "A boss who gets tired and shows it, who can't put in a series of twenty-hour days when necessary, who is seen to lose his edge in a physically wearing, long-drawn-out series of negotiations, is not the boss who is going to gain a great deal of respect."

- *It counteracts the biochemical effects of stress.* When Neanderthal man came face to face with a saber-toothed tiger in the primeval forests, his body was immediately prepared for action. His pulse raced, his blood pressure soared and a sudden outpouring of the stress hormones adrenaline and noradrenaline released into his bloodstream a flow of sugar and fatty acids, which are the fuels of muscular activity. He was ready for flight or fight. The same changes occur today when a businessman suffers a rebuff at work or endures the frustrations of driving in congested rush-hour traffic. But generally the atavistic stress response is wholly inappropriate. He is not going to run in terror from the monster which frightens him on the highway, or punch an irritating co-worker on the nose. So the tension and the biochemical changes persist. Since the fatty acids are not burned up by a sudden burst of muscular activity, they tend to be deposited in the blood vessel walls where they form the basis of atherosclerosis and coronary disease. As Dr. Malcolm Carruthers writes in *The Western Way of Death,* "The combination of a high level of emotional activity, together with a low level of physical activity, deranges body chemistry and is the major cause of heart disease." To compensate for this, people who are under stress should exercise regularly. This was recognized over two thousand years ago by Plato, who said: "Anyone engaged in mathematics or any other strenuous intellectual pursuit should also exercise his body and take part in physical training."

- *It reduces the risk of psychological illness.* Studies show that there is a close correlation between mental health and physical fitness. Dr. Lloyd Appleton of West Point assessed the physical condition of a large group of the Academy's cadets and found that psychological symptoms diminished as fitness increased. He encountered no psychiatric problems whatsoever in the very fittest students, whereas psychiatric discharges had to be given to nearly thirteen percent of cadets with the lowest fitness ratings.

Pavlov also noticed that lowered health hastened the breakdown of dogs subjected to experimental stress, and when political prisoners today are being prepared for brainwashing, they are always softened up first by a process of physical debilitation. If we have a heavy work load and want to cope without suffering undue stress, we must find time to maintain our physical health.

Professor Hans Eysenck, of the Institute of Psychiatry, London, is a prolific research worker, broadcaster and author, yet he finds time to play one or two hours of tennis or squash every lunch time. "How the mind behaves depends on the body," he says. "If I don't play for two or three days my mind doesn't work well, I'm struggling in my work and feel unhappy."

It would be wrong of course to suggest that fitness is simply a matter of getting adequate exercise. The secret of good health lies in the establishment of proper habits. There is no need to be a fitness fanatic, but since we have to eat we may as well learn to eat properly. As we need and want to work we may as well cultivate the art of working with maximum efficiency and ease. And while we are about it, we might also develop the habit of walking correctly and of using our eyes properly.

Hans Selye showed, for example, that a diet rich in salt tends to potentiate the harmful effects of stress. There is also clinical evidence that an excess of salt predisposes to high blood pressure. Cultures with a low intake of salt, like the Eskimos, suffer little hypertension, while those who use copious quantities of salt to preserve or season their food, like the Japanese, frequently succumb to high blood pressure. It is prudent therefore for people in stressful occupations to limit their intake of salt. It is also advisable for them to take increased quantities of vitamin C, since this important vitamin is metabolised more rapidly when we are under stress. Tests conducted in one penitentiary showed that prisoners used up twice as much vitamin C when they were under stress.

Masked food allergies can also place considerable strain on the body's powers of adaptation and in this way potentiate the harmful effect of environmental stress. The common offenders are milk, eggs, coffee and white flour. A food allergy can be suspected if after eating certain foods your pulse starts to race, and you feel excessively tired, muddleheaded, nauseous and giddy. In the opinion of Dr. Richard Mackarness, head of the food allergy clinic at Park Prewett Hospital, Basingstoke, England, as much as one-third of mental illness may be caused by specific dietary allergies. The treatment naturally rests on the identification and avoidance of the offending food.

The person who wishes to lessen the impact of stress and maintain his health and working efficiency needs to develop the habit of eating wisely. But then this applies to every other facet of our lives. By forty we are, in the words of psychologist William James, a "bundle of habits." If these habits of eating, drinking, sleeping and exercising are sound, our health will be strong and we will possess a high degree of stress tolerance.

Part II
THE ORIGIN OF STRESS

4
THE SPICE OF LIFE

Variety is the spice of life, too much variety the kiss of death. In the past a man's working day provided the stimulus of constant change. To survive, he had to act as hunter, carpenter, gardener, mechanic and herbalist. No two days were quite alike. His work was hard, but rarely boring. Now, with the introduction of mechanization and techniques of mass production, the work of many men has become soft and stultifying in its monotonous routine. The man who once pitted his wits against the elements and exercised his skills tracking game, building log cabins and cultivating crops, is now destined to spend a lifetime performing trivial, repetitive tasks. Day after day, he may be asked to do no more than drill four holes into a wooden frame, the same four holes drilled into identical frames, brought to him at regular thirty-second intervals by a conveyor belt whose speed never varies. Only *homo sapiens* could invent and impose so refined a form of torture and maintain a system which is so patently inhumane, injurious and inefficient.

To work at peak efficiency we all need a certain optimum level of novelty and change. Pavlov showed that an animal's natural response to a new stimulus is one of increased alertness and arousal. This keeps them "on the ball." With insufficient variety they become bored and apathetic. Most animals enjoy the stimulus of change and show a natural curiosity. Experiments have shown that if rats are given the choice of entering one of the two arms of a Y-shaped maze, they will invariably choose the arm which offers them a degree of novelty or change. Housewives bored by the endless repetition of routine household chores will perk themselves up by investing in an exotic new hairstyle; apathetic schoolchildren will raise their adrenaline levels by performing elaborate dares; middle-aged businessmen will break the monotony of their humdrum office lives by waging a brief but nevertheless stimulating, affair with a young secretary.

Organizations intent on following a policy of job enrichment must pay close attention to the need of their staff for regular change. The executive allowed to stay too long in one position will often dig a rut so deep that he is totally lost from view; and the factory worker ground down by years of soul-destroying repetitive work will understandably come to value his job less than his exciting new hobby, and wage increases alone will be powerless to recapture his lost enthusiasm. Volvo, the Swedish car manufacturers, has introduced a program of job rotation into its upholstery shop at Torsalanda, and has found that with careful managerial control it is possible to inject variety into routine manual work without any loss of productivity. This helps prevent the boredom which must inevitably arise when an increasingly educated work force is required to perform mundane, facile jobs.

To those fatigued by the routine sameness of their work, a change can be as good as a rest. Too much change, however, is potentially damaging, particularly if it is introduced with excessive haste. To minimize disruption and limit social discord, industrial innovations should be introduced slowly, and only after full consultation with all concerned. Changes of great magnitude need to be gradually introduced. Nature provides us with a perfect example in this respect. She colors our world with endless variety— the turn of the seasons, the transition from night to day, the progressive stages of human growth—but allows none of these changes to be introduced so abruptly that they strain our powers of adaptation. As Dickens wrote; "Nature gives to every time and season beauties of its own; and from morning to night, as from the cradle to the grave, is but a succession of changes so gentle and easy that we can scarcely mark their progress." She provides a transitional period of several years for women to accommodate to the hormonal changes of menopause, and a similar time for youngsters to acclimatize to the physiological changes and emotional crises of puberty.

Strain also occurs when an excess of change is allowed to disturb the routine order of our lives. In the twentieth century there has been a rapid acceleration in the rate of change, and in 1970 Alvin Toffler coined the term *future shock* "to describe the shattering stress and disorientation that we induce in individuals by subjecting them to too much change in too short a time." In graphic terms he illustrated the impact of the new technology on our lives. Dividing the last 50,000 years of man's existence into 800 lifetimes of approximately sixty-two years, he pointed out that the first 650 generations of man lived in caves. Only in the last 70 lifetimes has it been possible to transmit wisdom from one age to another through the medium of the written word; only in the last two has it been possible to measure time with any degree of accuracy; and only in the last two have we had the benefit of the electric motor. Moreover, he added, "The overwhelming majority of all the material goods we use today have been developed within the present, the 800th, lifetime." So we have achieved a dizzying rate of change, not by an orderly process of biological evolution, but by the frenzied maelstrom of technological revolution. This has brought material wealth, often at the cost of psychological impoverishment. At the same time our psychic poise has been disturbed by a profound degree of social change. At one time man had no doubt about his place in society. His life was spent in one homogeneous environment, he enjoyed the security of firmly established roots and did not suffer the stress of constant moves. If he was raised a carpenter, he most probably lived and died a carpenter. He did not normally strive to exchange his lot with that of a banker, landowner or property developer. He knew his role as employee, husband and father and experienced few of the identity crises and role conflicts endemic in today's society where the culturally accepted relationships between parents and children, employers and employees, men and women are constantly changing. If he was a merchant, he could safely conduct his business as his father and grandfather had done before him. If trading conditions altered they did so only gradually; there were no rapid upheavals in tax laws, interest rates, export regulations, or trade union agreements. Life was stable and orderly. Today we live in a transient age where change is the order of the day: a highway where there used to be country fields, girls in boys' clothing, a hamburger stand where there once was the corner grocery store. For many this degree of change is too great to tolerate.

Sickness is frequently a failure of adaptation. This was recognized by Hippocrates, who said: "It is changes that are chiefly responsible for diseases." This is seen in industry where, according to Dr. D.S.F. Robertson, an English Industrial Medical Officer, "It is during the period of adaptation after starting work in a new job or under new supervision, accepting new responsibilities and promotion or returning to work after a long absence (whatever the cause of the absence), that the individual is found with the greatest problem of psychological adaptation and consequently is most likely to succumb to psychological breakdown." The same fate overtakes society at large, for as Professor Dubos, Editor of the *Journal of Experimental Medicine*, has noted: "In Europe and America, all periods of social upheaval have been accompanied by a marked increase of the incidence of disease." The ideal is to inject the right degree of variety into our lives to achieve maximum performance by steering a narrow course between the boredom of too little change and the exhaustion of too much. The optimum level of arousal varies considerably from individual to individual. Experimental studies have shown that anxious individuals require less stimulation to maintain their emotional poise and are naturally less adventurous and more readily threatened by unfamiliar tasks and situations.

Charles Darwin was the perfect example of a distinguished man who could tolerate little alteration in his normal, day-to-day routine. Even a visit from a friend or a small dinner party would make him physically sick. As he wrote in his *Life and Letters*: "I find most unfortunately for myself, that the excitement of breaking out of my most quiet routine so generally knocks me up, that I am unable to do scarcely anything while in London."

Successful entrepreneurs and business executives are generally made of sterner stuff and can happily tackle business meetings, travel and dinner parties without suffering any qualms. But even they are not immune to the effects of overwhelming change. Dr. Thomas Holmes, Professor of Psychiatry at the University of Washington, made a detailed study of the effects of change on our physical and mental well-being and discovered that "four out of every five people who have experienced many dramatic changes in their lives over the past year can expect a major illness within the next two years." With the help of Richard Rahe, then a medical student, he evolved a Social Readjustment Rating Scale which makes it possible to estimate the degree of adaptational stress we are suffering at any given time (see table). He found that while eighty percent of people with scores over 300 and fifty-three percent of people with scores in the 150–300 range became pathologically depressed, had heart attacks or suffered other forms of serious illness, these disorders occurred in only thirty-three percent of people with scores under 150. This research suggests that whenever possible we should limit the amount of change occurring during any one period of our lives.

Stress Value of Life Changes

Event	Score
Death of spouse	100
Divorce	73
Marital separation	65
Jail term	63
Death of close member of family	63
Personal injury or illness	53
Marriage	50

Fired from job	47
Marital reconciliation	45
Retirement	45
Change in health in member of family	44
Pregnancy	40
Sex difficulties	39
Gain of new family member	39
Change in financial state	38
Death of close friend	37
Change to different type of work	36
Change in number of arguments with spouse	35
Mortgage over $10,000	31
Foreclosure of mortgage or loan	30
Change of responsibility at work	29
Son or daughter leaves home	29
Trouble with in-laws	29
Wife beginning or stopping work	29
Outstanding personal achievement	28
Beginning or ending school	26
Revision of personal habits	24
Trouble with boss	23
Change in hours or conditions of work	20
Change in residence	20
Change in schools	20
Change in recreation	19
Change in social activities	18
Mortgage or loan less than $10,000	17
Change in sleeping habits	16
Change in number of family get-togethers	15
Change in eating habits	15
Vacation	13
Minor violations of the law	11

Steps can also be taken to limit the harmful effects of certain specific changes. Many executives, for example, make frequent changes in their homes and jobs. During his lifetime the average American moves about fourteen times. This involves the corporate gypsy in both losses and gains. He gains the advantage of a better job, but loses the company of some valued co-workers. He may take up residence in a splendid new home with a heated swimming pool, but parts company with his old golf club, neighbors and local dramatic society. On the Holmes/Rahe scale, allowing for his change of job, home, living conditions and mortgage, he may clock up a significant 100 points of change. This is enough to make him a potential candidate for one or another of the recognized stress diseases. The change will also have a profound effect upon his family, particularly his wife who will have to cope with decorating and furnishing a new home, forging new friendships, establishing new shopping patterns and building an entirely new social life. This can be a cause of considerable marital discord, and when a key executive is moved, far more attention should be paid to the needs of his wife and family. To limit the stress arising from a change of home and job it is advisable for a married executive to:

- Consult the family beforehand about the move, pointing out in particular its advantages in terms of advancement and growth.
- Subscribe in advance to the new local paper and study as much as possible about the history, attractions and amenities of the new area.
- Take the family on a weekend visit to the new town and discover the parks, golf clubs, sports centers, youth clubs, public library, churches and shopping centers.
- Try to plan for the continuity of family hobbies and activities by linking up with adult education institutes, sports clubs, dramatic societies and voluntary organizations.
- Arrange for visits of family friends, particularly the

Endeavor —старание

children's friends, to ease the trauma of initial separation.

- Endeavor as far as possible to maintain family rituals and traditions in the new setting.

Many executives also suffer the strain of frequent and rapid airplane trips. In Biblical times the fastest means of transportation was the camel caravan traveling at roughly 8 m.p.h. With the invention of the horse-drawn chariot in approximately 1600 B.C. it became possible to travel at 20 m.p.h., a pace which was not exceeded for well over 3,000 years. The early steam trains could muster a speed of no more than 13 m.p.h., and it was only the introduction of more efficient steam locomotives at the end of the nineteenth century which made it possible to travel at 100 m.p.h. Since then there has been a rapid increase in the speed of travel. By 1938 airplanes were capable of traveling at 400 m.p.h. and a few decades later space capsules were orbiting the earth at 18,000 m.p.h. This incredible increase in transport speeds has placed considerable strains on man's powers of adaptation, giving rise to a condition known popularly as "jet lag," or more accurately as "time-zone fatigue." This produces symptoms of fatigue, insomnia, irritability, digestive disorder, delayed reaction times and impaired judgment. Under its influence we think and act more slowly than usual. The condition arises, not because we are traveling long distances at rapid speeds, but because we upset the orderly working of our internal clock mechanisms. Identical changes occur in shift workers and can be produced experimentally by artificially turning night into day. All living organisms from cabbages to kings are geared to a twenty-four-hour day. Humans are no exception and show a regular diurnal rhythm in most of their bodily functions. Sleep pattern, body temperature, blood pressure, rate of kidney flow, and blood sugar level all show a consistent rise and fall during the twenty-four hours. Rapid latitudinal travel upsets this careful synchronization, with frequently disturbing results. The kidneys, for example, are conveniently scheduled to produce the maximum flow of urine by day, and considerably less by night. But the traveler who makes a rapid east-west flight turns night into day and so is liable to suffer the inconvenience of having to get up several times during the night to empty a bladder which is still working on the old time schedule. Extensive tests made on a group of travelers flying on a round trip between San Francisco and London showed that they suffered a twenty percent drop in alertness and a fifteen to twenty-five percent reduction in concentration after their flights. The disturbance was more pronounced, and took longer to resolve, on the eastward leg of the flight, a phenomenon for which there is at present no obvious explanation. Some physical weakness may also be experienced after a long flight, for studies have shown that time-zone fatigue produces a five to seven percent reduction in muscular strength. This small drop may be of little importance if the traveler's only exertion on arrival is to turn off the light in his hotel bedroom, but if he happens to have a weak heart, and needs to carry a suitcase up a flight of stairs, even a slight decline in the strength of his myocardial muscles could be critical. Changes like these subject the body to a considerable degree of stress, as was confirmed when passengers and crew flying by Concorde from Buenos Aires to London were subjected to biochemical tests. These showed a marked elevation in the level of circulating stress hormones—adrenaline, noradrenaline and cortisol—which did not return to normal until two days after the flight. There is even a possibility that frequent jet travel may shorten our life expectancy for it has been found that rats subjected to a weekly inversion of their night-day cycle suffer an average six percent decrease in their life span.

Several measures can be adopted to reduce the negative effects of rapid time-zone travel:

- *Recognize the problem.* The effects of jet lag are frequently noticed by everyone but the traveler himself, who, though tired and irritable, struggles to keep himself going with whiskey, cigars and coffee. These stimulants merely aggravate a problem which basically only time can cure. It takes the body at least six days to adjust fully to east- or west-bound flights of four or more hours' duration, and if individuals will not make the necessary allowance for this, companies must lay down definite guidelines for them to follow. Executives should neither be expected nor allowed to make important decisions immediately after a long journey. The World Bank has said: "Our executives are adults and should be able to decide for themselves whether to take a rest or not." Unfortunately experience shows that most executives if left to their own devices do not make adequate provision for the effect of jet fatigue. In England, Imperial Chemical Industries advise their executives to allow at least twenty-four hours for acclimatization after a flight involving time-zone transit. Ideally a longer period should be allowed for elderly executives who take longer to adapt, and particularly to reestablish their normal pattern of sleep.

- *Remain synchronized to home time.* On short trips try as far as possible to maintain a routine of eating and sleeping synchronized to home time. If necessary wear two watches, one set to local time, the other to home time. On longer journeys make a gradual readjustment in eating and sleeping patterns, moving them forward or back by no more than an hour a day. This is the policy adopted by Russian pilots on the Moscow-Havana run who throughout their stay in Cuba adhere to base time and eat breakfast at midnight, supper at noon and retire to bed at 3:00 A.M. This policy would be made easier if every international airport had at least one "time-lock" hotel, where aircraft passengers and crew could be maintained within the time schedules of their own countries.

- *Avoid overeating* and deviate as little as possible from the normal patterns of eating and drinking, even if this means refusing free meals and drinks during the flight and shunning on arrival the curried prawns and other exotic local delicacies.

- *Drink plenty of water during the flight,* for some of the symptoms of jet lag are caused by dehydration which occurs when the body is exposed to the low humidity and pressure within the cabin of a modern jet. As alcohol is a diuretic and encourages the loss of fluid from the body, this is another reason for avoiding heavy drinking during a long flight.

- *Take some form of exercise during the trip.* Much of the fatigue of jet travel, like the lethargy experienced at the end of the Christmas festivities, is the result of indolence and overindulgence in food and drink. In 1976 Lufthansa, the West German national airline, tried to reduce flight fatigue by offering passengers a program of broadcast exercises which they could perform in their seats. A sensible alternative is to combine a visit to the toilet with a few seconds' vigorous calisthenics.

- *Whenever possible take a trans-polar flight* in preference to one of the regular circumferential routes. Since flights along the lines of longitude do not cross any time-zones, they do not cause any disturbance of the body's internal clock mechanism.

- *Travel in company if possible.* Research has shown that, for reasons that are not clear, groups of travelers are less affected by fatigue than solo passengers.

The executive who wishes to work at maximum efficiency and minimal strain must, among other things, cultivate the delicate art of injecting into his life sufficient variety to provide the stimulus of novelty, challenge and fresh experience without allowing himself to be overloaded at any one time with an excess of bewildering change. His health depends upon his skill in achieving the required balance, for as Alvin Toffler wrote, "Some level of change is as vital to health as too much change is damaging." Fortunately, there are several practical steps which can be taken to assist the body's adaptation to the frequently rapid changes of modern business life.

- *Train for change.* We can increase our powers of adaptation by systematically training the body to cope with upheavals in our normal routine. We can vaccinate our bodies against future shock by exposing them frequently to small doses of change. The creature of rigid habits and strict conformity can easily be overcome by even a trivial change in office routine. To achieve flexibility we must practice flexibility. Routines need occasionally to be turned upside-down. At times we should catch an earlier train to work, read a different newspaper, vacation in the winter instead of in the summer, take up a new hobby, grow a beard or get up at dawn and take a long walk before breakfast. This provides both an immediate tonic and a long-term protection against the time when change is thrust upon us.

- *Try whenever possible to anticipate change* and forestall its shock effect. We recognize the importance of preparing for retirement, and need to use equal foresight in preparing for all the other major changes in our lives. When change is introduced into industry it should be handled in a way that provides full consultation with all those involved, and entails a minimum disruption of their individual and group life. As the National Research Council concluded in its 1941 report *Fatigue of Workers and Its Relation to Industrial Problems*: "The successful management of any human enterprise depends largely upon the ability to introduce more efficient methods without disrupting in the process the social foundation on which collaboration is based."

- *Control the rate and volume of change.* The man who has recently been widowed is well advised to allow some months to pass before he moves and loses the support and company of his old friends. The executive whose twenty-year-old marriage has just ended in divorce should give himself time to adjust before he takes on the responsibility of a new job. As Toffler says, "If we are to avoid a massive adaptational breakdown, we must learn to control the rate of change not only in our personal affairs but in society at large." Our politicians could help the nation achieve this end by providing the necessary framework of social and economic stability. Many of the small businessmen in Great Britain were overwhelmed by the sudden introduction of currency decimalization, value-added tax and the metric system. Changes of this magnitude should, whenever possible, be introduced more gradually over a longer period of time.

- *Endeavor to see change in its historical perspective.* Even a cursory knowledge of history is enough to show that, while we may be living through an era of tumultuous change, there is an underlying bedrock of permanence, a reassuring continuity. As Alphonse Karr observed: *"Plus ça change, plus c'est la même chose"* (The more things change, the more they are the same). The wind of change merely ruffles the leaves of time, while the tree of life itself remains firmly rooted in eternity. Most of the world's leaders have shown a passionate interest in history and from this they have drawn comfort and strength. The more we study the upheavals of the past the better we are able to understand and handle the changes of the present. As the historian G. M. Trevelyan observes: "The present is always taking us by surprise, because we do not sufficiently know and consider the past."

- *Establish stability zones.* During times of rapid change it is helpful to retreat into the comfort and security of familiar situations and routines. Just as a child sleeping for the first time in a strange bed will insist on the company of a well-loved teddy bear, so the adult victim of oppressive change can derive comfort from reading a well-loved book, puttering in the garden in an old pair of jeans, or having a dinner party with old school friends. Ethologists have shown that all animals feel most secure when they are on home territory. Planarium worms take twice as long to settle down and start to eat in unfamiliar environments as they do in their native feeding grounds, and a study of the graceful Uganda kob shows that in battles waged on unfamiliar ground it is the interloper who is virtually always defeated. Elephants subjected to unusual shocks, like the sounding of a motor horn, have been known to die of a heart attack; but this is less likely to happen if they are in familiar surroundings and accompanied by other members of their herd.

We need to develop areas of stability in our lives, emotional foxholes into which we can retreat when the battle grows too fierce. The comfort of a day's trout fishing in the country, or maybe an hour of two operating the model train in the attic. Above all else, perhaps, the businessman's home must become his castle, a nest where he can retire from the hustle and feel secure and inviolable.

5

THE SKY'S THE LIMIT

Ours is an achievement-orientated society. From a very early age we are encouraged to strive for bigger and better things. We are fascinated by superlatives—by best-selling novels, top-ten songs, the town's most beautiful baby and the world's richest man. Whatever we have we want a little more. The teenage boy craves another few inches in height, his older brother a faster car, his mother a larger bust. In business we have adopted the Protestant ethic, which proclaims the virtues of hard work, thrift and competitive struggle. "It's the game that matters," we tell our opponents in sport and business, but we all know it is winning that counts. Life has no time for failures and it recognizes no such thing as a "good" loser. Even the founders of the Olympic games in 776 B.C. placed little or no emphasis on participation for its own sake, and no prizes whatsoever were offered to the athletes who came second or third. It was the winner's wreath alone that mattered. We need to hitch our wagon to a star if we are to achieve excellence in commerce, art and sport. As Lord Lytton, a nineteenth-century author, said, "The man who succeeds above his fellows is the one who early in life clearly discerns his object and toward that object habitually directs his powers." Unfortunately this steadfast craving can also make him avaricious, selfish and sick. This disadvantage was clearly appreciated by I. G. Wyllie, who in his study of *The Self-Made Man in America* said: "The ambition to succeed may be, and always ought to be, a laudable one. It is the ambition of every parent for his child. It is emphatically an American ambition: at once the national vice and the national virtue. It is the mainspring of activity; the driving wheel of industry; the spur to intellectual and moral progress. It gives the individual energy; the nation push. It makes the difference between a people that are a stream and a people that are a pool; between America and China. It makes us at once active and restless; industrious and overworked; generous and greedy."

Well-meaning attempts have been made by many educationalists to curb the competitive spirit, but hard as they try to eliminate it from the classroom, it reemerges in the playground in the form of highly competitive games which children invariably choose to play when left to their own devices. A reasonable degree of ambition and competitiveness is natural in a child, and should be fostered as the foundation of success and the bulwark of self-esteem. Care must be taken, however, to see that unrealized ambitions do not lead to sickness and despair. Many of the youngsters encouraged to strive for academic standards above their natural abilities fall by the wayside, some take drugs, others hit the bottle, attempt suicide, develop asthma or express a variety of other stress symptoms. The overambitious businessman may suffer an early heart attack. Personality profiles show that the man prone to a heart attack "commonly possesses an ambitious, driving nature and exhibits a consistent tendency toward compulsive striving, self-discipline and hard work. He frequently sets herculean tasks for himself, exceeding his normal capacity and tempo, minimizing warning signals and neglecting prudent rules of health." It is probably this factor, rather than his heavy smoking or cholesterol-rich diet, which determines the likelihood of a coronary attack. The Japanese male has always had a much lower rate of coronary disease than his American counterpart. This difference was for many years attributed to his diet, which, with its preponderance of fish and rice, had a low content of animal fat. Recent research suggests that this dietary discrepancy is probably of only slight significance. More important is the traditional Japanese way of life, which minimizes the harmful effects of competition by maintaining a strict social hierarchy in which everyone knows his or her place, and in which competition is recognized as a group activity rather than a lonely personal struggle. Certainly there is little coronary disease among Japanese men working in San Francisco who have adopted the American diet and smoking patterns but retained the Japanese way of life. The rates, however, are two-and-a-half times higher for those who have made a moderate transition to a Western way of life, and five times higher for those who have immersed themselves completely in the highly competitive American way of life.

High competitiveness can also be a cause of nervous breakdown, anxiety, and depressive illness. Psychiatrists have noted that elation is generally related to success, while depression tends to follow a period of actual or considered failure. Psychologists also recognize a state they call "achievement anxiety," a state brought on by a pervasive fear of failure. In laboratory experiments they have induced states of anxiety by motivating people to complete a series of puzzles successfully, then providing them with problems which cannot be solved. In parallel experiments they induced a state of anxiety in volunteers by allowing them to complete a series of mathematical problems, then falsely informing them that they had failed. But it is not only the psychologists' guinea pigs who experience the pangs of thwarted ambition or the depression of real or imagined failure. This sad state overtakes many men in their middle years, when they reach a watershed in their lives and are forced to accept the painful fact that they will never achieve their life's long-standing hopes and cherished ambitions. Because of its similarity to the emotional changes experienced by women during the change of life, this crisis is often referred to as the male menopause, but there are no equivalent hormonal changes. The condition is more aptly referred to in German as the *Torschlusspanik* (the panic of the closing doors). Professor Ken Rogers, Professor of Psychiatry at the New Jersey College of Medicine and Dentistry, has made a detailed study of the crisis which occurs in the lives of many middle-aged American and British males, and has found that in the fourth decade of their lives many men "stated explicitly that they felt their careers and their entire lives had reached some sort of plateau . . . that life did not hold out any excitement or opportunities for major satisfactions." A crisis like this can occur at any time during an executive's life. To prevent its occurring it is necessary to:

- *Set realistic goals.* Management by objectives is a well-established managerial technique, but the same principles should be applied to the setting of personal targets. These need to be clearly defined and realistic. A skilled cabinet maker would find it difficult to construct a liquor cabinet without a set of detailed plans. Equally an executive cannot achieve his life's aim unless he has a definite blueprint to follow. When Alice asked the Cheshire Cat, "Would you tell me please, which way I ought to go from here?" the cat quite sensibly replied, "That depends a good deal on where you want to go." We need to know first of all the goal, and then the steps which need to be taken to achieve the goal. These subsidiary targets need to be set realistically. If we want to be an Olympic high jumper and can as yet manage to clear a height of only five feet two inches, it would be unrealistic to aim to jump seven feet by the end of the year. In the same way if an average bowler sets the goal of scoring six strikes out of every ten possible he would suffer repeated disappointment and soon give up the game. But the more realistic goal of scoring a minimum of one strike out of every ten, would spur him to increase his accuracy and skill. As Norman Maier, Professor of Psychology at the University of Michigan, has said: "A person who is well adjusted to his work has the proper balance between ability and level of aspiration." The frequent failure of executives to select clear and realistic goals for themselves is a common cause of stress and dissipated talent and skill. We must try to liberate ourselves from desires we know we cannot satisfy. The art is to make a bouquet with the flowers within our grasp.

- *Establish "personal" targets.* The ideal is to set our own goals and travel at our own pace to achieve them. Too many people unquestioningly accept the aspirations of their friends or the stimulated desires of advertising. "Keeping up with the Joneses" is commendable only when we genuinely want what the Joneses have got. In today's society we often stimulate desires which cannot then be satisfied. A middle-aged business man in a strange city visits a "Playboy" club, sees the alluring appeal of his Bunny hostess, but knows he cannot touch. In the same way a young executive is sent to a staff training college to learn the delights and skills of higher managerial control, only to return to his old job as head of the typing pool. Frustration is the inevitable result. The wise executive sets his own goals, competes against himself and his past achievements, and does not allow desires to be stimulated that he knows he cannot satisfy.

- *Avoid conflicting goals.* It is advisable to establish one's priorities by devising a hierarchy of goals, never forgetting to include in the scheme of things an answer to the fundamental question "What is the ultimate purpose of my life?" Many executives say they place health, happiness and the welfare of their family before their loyalty to their company. Then they take a job which removes them from their families for many months of the year, causes them endless frustration and possibly drives them to an early grave. We often suffer short-term privations for what we imagine will be the long-term good, but frequently the tomorrows we are working for never arrive. It is often necessary to compromise between short- and long-term goals. For example, if our aim is to achieve the maximum return on capital invested prior to getting a public quotation it might be advisable to make a drastic reduction in stocks and prune expenditure on research and development programs, but neither policy would be in the long-term interests of the company. Achieving a compromise between long- and short-term aims is never simple, but it is made much easier if our goals are clearly defined. We often struggle to acquire more of the world's material wealth, a goal which may have been realistic when we were penurious students but which has far less purpose when we are well-fed, well-housed, secure adults. Most executives when questioned place a relatively low priority on income as a source of primary satisfaction. When management consultants Booz, Allen and Hamilton asked 422 executives why they had changed their jobs they received the following replies: to obtain a bigger job with more responsibility; because of a disagreement with the management policies of the previous firm; because advancement had been blocked; or because they felt in need of a change. The desire to get more income was relegated to seventh place in the list. Yet many successful men make it an unquestioned goal to acquire more and more money, even though they know that in practice they can only eat three meals a day, wear one suit and occupy one home. And the more they amass the more they have to worry about.

The world-famous ethologist Hans Hass sees countless problems for the wealth-bound man. "If a man augments his organizational system with too much property, with too many artificially acquired organs, time becomes too short for him to exploit all the opportunities they offer, and they turn against him. They make certain demands on him, coercing, compelling, tempting; the controlling cerebral structures war against one another and make the man restless and discontented despite his wealth." The man who buys shares of stock to give himself security also acquires a large measure of insecurity for the value of shares can go down as well as up.

- *Whenever possible choose corporate goals* rather than individual goals. In primitive societies competition was primarily between groups rather than individuals. A group of Indian hunters teamed up to capture a buffalo, the warriors from an Ibos village combined to ward off the attack of a marauding band of neighboring tribesmen. In today's society competition is chiefly between individuals. We meet only as competitors for a job; as buyers and sellers, antagonists in the marketplace. Our adherence to the Protestant work ethic involves us in a continual, undisciplined rat race, where success is seen as the reward of aggressive struggle rather than peaceful cooperation. To win means to get the better of someone else in bedroom, boardroom or battlefield. To the winner goes the temporary crown, to the loser the wooden spoon of failure and an accompanying loss of self-esteem. Undoubtedly there is a place for the lone maverick and a time when individual assertion and aggressiveness is necessary to achieve our goals, but the maintenance of an unnecessarily high level of competition is damaging for the individual, the corporation for which he works, and for society itself. The gradual realization of this inherent defect in the Protestant work ethic has led to a revolt against aggressive individualism. In its place there have sprung up numerous corporate endeavors—communes, housing associations, parent-teacher associations, encounter groups and large multi-national corporations. The tough Protestant ethic is being balanced by a more gentle "social ethic," the major propositions of which are, according to William Whyte: "A belief in the group as the source of creativity; a belief in 'belongingness' as the ultimate need of the individual; and a belief in the application of science to achieve the belongingness." The conflict between these schools of thought will be discussed at greater length in Chapter 11.

- *Do not try too hard.* Performance can deteriorate under the pressure of excessive strain. The over-zealous golfer slices his drive; the over-eager job hunter stammers through his interview; the mind of the student, desperately anxious to pass an examination, goes blank the moment he reads the test paper. Excessive striving can be self-defeating, a fact confirmed by experiments carried out by Professor Jerome Bruner of Harvard University. He gave two groups of rats a complicated maze to solve in order to reach a supply of food, and found that whereas mildly hungry rats solved the maze in about six tries, those who hadn't eaten for thirty-six hours, in their overeagerness to satisfy their hunger, took more than twenty tries.

- *Avoid rigidity.* Stress frequently arises when attempts are made to uphold high standards under adverse conditions. The housewife worries herself into a migraine attack when she cannot maintain a scrupulously tidy home during the visit of her three unruly grandchildren; an accountant triggers off another gastric ulcer simply because he is behind schedule with his work at a time when his secretary is away sick, his junior partner on vacation and he's trying in the evenings to produce a play for the local amateur drama group. Flexible goals are invaluable guidelines. Inflexible goals can be crippling fetters. We must not drive so relentlessly forward that we cannot stop to smell the roses by the wayside. We must achieve resting points of contentment in our lives, for the good life exists only when we stop wanting a better one. Cineas the philosopher once asked Pyrrhus, King of Epirus, what he would do when he had conquered Italy. "I will conquer Sicily." "And after Sicily?" "Then Africa." "And after you have conquered the world?" "Then I will take my ease and be merry." "In that case," said Cineas, "why can you not take your ease and be merry now?" The desire to enjoy greater prosperity should not prevent us from enjoying the prosperity we have already achieved, nor should we feel unduly guilty about doing so. To keep the wheels of industry turning we need to spend as well as to save, to be idle as well as to work. Unfortunately we often feel guilty about enjoying our new-found prosperity. According to Dr. Ernest Dichter, the eminent motivational researcher, one of the basic problems of this newly acquired material prosperity "is to give people the sanction and justification to enjoy it and to demonstrate that the hedonistic approach to life is a moral, not an immoral one."

- *Do not be deterred by failure*. It is hard to conceive a life without occasional setbacks. Most of the world's successful people have at one time considered themselves failures. As William James said, "Take the happiest man, the one most envied by the world, and in nine cases out of ten his inmost consciousness is one of failure. Either his ideals in the line of his achievements are pitched far higher than the achievements themselves, or else he has secret ideals of which the world knows nothing, and in regard to which he inwardly knows himself to be found wanting." We must accept the occasional reverse as one of the inescapable facts of life, and in seeking to achieve our goals, must not be deterred by an overwhelming fear of failure. To fail in itself is not a sin; failure to attempt is the only indictable crime.

One man made a study of the personality traits of successful men and found that they had one characteristic in common—persistence. Typical of the group was the man who failed in business in '31, was defeated in politics in '32, failed again in business in '34, had a nervous breakdown in '41, and failed to receive his party's nomination for Congress in '43. That man was Abraham Lincoln, who in his early days may have been written off by many as a perennial loser, but who overcame his early setbacks to become one of the greatest Presidents of the United States. As Lincoln proved, you are defeated only when you stop trying.

6

THE FINAL STRAW

Most people if asked to give reasons for the increasing strain of modern life would lay a large measure of blame on the "pressure of work." We are constantly struggling to force a ton of work into a bushel of time and have the perpetual task of trying to satisfy an increasing number of bosses, bureaucrats, employees and union officials. One looks back with envy on the more leisurely days when a businessman could find time to solve *The New York Times* crossword puzzle over his morning coffee, and after lunch at the club could while away the afternoon hours checking his personal portfolio of stocks as he sipped a cup or two of coffee. It was a restful life enjoyed by even the heads of state: an era of enviable ease when Theodore Roosevelt could reasonably hope to finish his Presidential work by midday and spend the afternoon playing with his children, and when Calvin Coolidge could settle down each night to an assured twelve hours' sleep. Since then the pressures of political life have steadily increased. When announcing his retirement from the rigors of high political office Harold Wilson gave some indication of the workload placed on a modern political executive. In nearly eight years as Prime Minister he claimed to have presided over 472 cabinet meetings, answered more than 12,000 parliamentary questions, read at least 500 documents each weekend and given an annual total of well over 100 speeches to "political and other" meetings. During that time, "apart from quite generous holidays," he had worked seven days a week and twelve to fourteen hours a day.

Work schedules of this nature can be maintained indefinitely providing the work is rewarding. Thomas Edison, the great inventor of the phonograph, incandescent lamp and over a thousand other devices, normally worked an eighteen-hour day and frequently took his few hours of sleep in his laboratory to avoid unnecessary curtailment of his work. Yet at the end of his long and successful life he could honestly say, "I never did a day's work in my life; it was all fun." Hard work is not the killer it is often thought to be, and some of the world's most prolific workers—Pablo Casals, Winston Churchill, Albert Schweitzer, Toscanini, Pablo Picasso, Charles de Gaulle and Konrad Adenauer—have lived to a ripe old age. Hard creative work of this kind can be a tonic and elixir. Dr. Hans Selye was so fascinated by the excitement of medical research as a young student that he established the habit of getting up at 4 A.M. and working through until 6 P.M. His mother warned him that if he continued at this hectic pace he was heading for a nervous breakdown, and friends advised him, "You should work to live, not live to work." Fifty years later Selye was still maintaining the same schedule of working from 4 A.M. to 6 P.M. and still thoroughly enjoying life. As he said: "To function normally, man *needs* work as he needs air, food, sleep, social contacts or sex."

Problems generally arise only when work is unsatisfying, frustrating, monotonous, and unsuccessful, or indulged in merely as a matter of obsessive routine. In Victorian England the greatest sin was not cruelty, gluttony, depravity or greed, but idleness. Children, from the moment they were old enough to read the inspirational works of Samuel Smiles and Lord Avebury, had drummed into them the principles of self-denial, hard work and thrift. Parents urged them to "try harder." School reports carried the awful warning: "Must show greater diligence." They worked to support the growth of the burgeoning Victorian economy, and industry became the path to personal salvation. This carefully instilled Protestant work ethic helped to make the Victorian age an era of unprecedented prosperity and growth. The principle is less forcibly held today, but remains a powerful regulator of human behavior and activity. We work because we are afraid to enjoy the fruits of idleness. We fill our days because we have a pathological need to assert our importance, or because we derive satisfaction within the impersonal bounds of our working situation which we cannot obtain in our close personal relationships. We become as surely addicted to work as others became addicted to alcohol and drugs. Wayne E. Oates, Professor of Religion at Southern Baptist Theological College, Louisville, Kentucky, clearly describes the condition in his book *Confessions of a Workaholic*. He was obsessed by "the uncontrollable urge to work incessantly," but realized the fact only when his five-year-old son jokingly tried to make an appointment to see him. The workaholic can be recognized, says Oates, because he "drops out of the human community"; eats, drinks and sleeps his job; is "merciless in his demands upon himself for peak performance," and unable to tell the difference between loyalty to his job and "compulsive overcommitment." Overwork of this order is invariably self-imposed, and though it may be undertaken for the highest possible motives it invariably leads to inefficiency and ill health.

Henry Ford I, after pushing his workers to the limit, was forced to admit that "we would have had our model A car in production six months sooner if I had forbidden my engineers to work on Sunday. It took all week to straighten out the mistakes they made on the day they should have rested." Similar effects were observed in Great Britain during the war, when under the threat of imminent invasion after the Dunkirk evacuation the average working week in munition factories was increased from fifty-six to sixty-nine and a half hours. To begin with there was a ten percent rise in output, but thereafter productivity declined as absenteeism, sickness and accidents soared. Fatigue also sets in if we struggle too long at mental tasks such as reciting the alphabet backwards, multiplying three-digit numbers in our head or memorizing complicated word sequences. Laboratory experiments have shown that if we work too long at these tasks, our problem-solving time can increase by 500 percent. When working under these pressures we become less efficient and also more prone to stress disease. Experiments conducted by Dr. Lennart Levi at the Laboratory for Clinical Stress Research in Stockholm have shown that when invoice clerks are encouraged to work above their normal rate by a system of incentive bonuses they suffer increased fatigue, greater physical discomfort and a marked rise in their output of stress hormones. Similar changes are seen in accountants, who can show a doubling in the level of cholesterol circulating in their blood, and a corresponding decrease in their blood coagulation time, during the hectic days leading up to the end of the tax year when they may be forced to work a seventy-hour week. Changes such as these make the overtaxed worker a potential candidate for stress disease. Even the toughest, most phlegmatic characters will eventually succumb to the harmful effects of repeated strain. Caesar's hand-picked Eagle-bearers were among the finest soldiers of the ancient world, and yet even these hardened campaigners broke down occasionally under the stress of thirteen years' continuous campaigning in Gaul. Every war produces its toll of sufferers from battle fatigue, and Dr. Roy Swank, after a study of 5,000 cases arising during the 1944 Normandy campaign, said that "all normal men eventually suffer combat exhaustion in prolonged, continuous and severe combat." The symptoms produced by this exhaustion— fatigue, irritability, impaired judgment and loss of confidence—are typical of prolonged struggles irrespective of whether they are waged on the battlefield or in an executive office. Unfortunately in the early stages these tell-tale symptoms often go unrecognized. Most harassed executives will deny that they are working too hard; that is just a fantasy concocted by their wives, doctors, family and friends. So they blithely push themselves on until the inevitable collapse comes and they are committed to the hospital with a heart attack, perforated ulcer or nervous breakdown. Providing they survive, only then do they take stock and endeavor to change their compulsive working habits. John Stuart Mill, whose education was so forced that he was reading Greek at the age of six, suffered a mental breakdown in his early twenties. He made a complete recovery and went on to accomplish prodigious amounts of work, but was so impressed by his experience that he advocated that everyone should overwork once in his life, so he could recognize and avoid the dangers later on. Better, surely, to learn the lesson without having to endure this painful personal experience. Overwork can be avoided by:

- *Learning to say no.* Most overwork is self-imposed. We find it hard to refuse the invitation to join the committee of the PTA. It is flattering to be asked to propose the toast to the guests at the Annual Rotarian dinner and challenging to be invited to organize the church's fund-raising campaign. But every task we accept adds to our overall burden. As Edwin C. Bliss says in *Getting Things Done*: "You cannot protect your priorities unless you learn to decline, tactfully but firmly, every request that does not contribute to your goal." It is often the accumulation of a multitude of relatively minor tasks which causes the ultimate damage. As Joseph L. Kearns, Group Medical Adviser to the J. Lyons Group of Companies in England, puts it: "It is more often the weight of minor stresses which produces breakdown than an intense specific stressor." It is the final straw that breaks the camel's back.

- *Do not overload your day with work.* A worker, like a car, should never be driven at full speed for long periods. We should aim to cruise through life, always keeping a little something in reserve for emergency use. Ideally the working day should be punctuated by frequent rest pauses. Physiological experiments have shown that both mental and physical work is best carried out in regular, alternating cycles of work and rest. In factories the introduction of official rest breaks (generally five minutes' break at the end of every hour's work) has led

to lessened fatigue, decreased absenteeism and production increases of from ten to thirteen percent.
This confirms the observation made by Thoreau:
"A really efficient laborer will be found not to
crowd his day with work."

- *Learn to delegate.* A long working day is very often
a sign of managerial inefficiency. It may stem from
an inability to delegate or a neurotic need to obtain
from obsessive work a repeated confirmation of our
ability and worth. We develop fantasies of omnipo-
tence, imagining that we alone can carry out the
allotted work. It is only when the "indispensable"
executive has a heart attack that he discovers just
how dispensable he is.

  Delegation confers a number of benefits. It gives
subordinates the freedom to work in their own way
without constant reference to the boss, frees managers to concentrate on the more important issues
that only they can handle, and makes them more
dispensable and therefore easier to promote.

  The main reason why managers fail to delegate
as much as they should is because they know that
they are accountable for the work of their subordinates and do not want to be blamed for any mistakes they might make. In the same way the chief
reason why subordinates are reluctant to take on
new responsibilities is that they do not want to
suffer criticism if they should fail. This means that
the process of delegation within an organization is
favored if the rewards for success are always made
greater than the punishment for failure.

- *Establish a system of priorities.* Find time to com-
pile a list of tasks to be tackled in order of their

urgency and importance. This can greatly reduce the burden of a heavy work load. It also acts as a reminder, removing the threat that something vital will be forgotten unless we consistently struggle to remember every job we have to do. Dr. Selye confessed to being an inveterate list maker. "There is a limit to how much you can burden your memory; and trying to remember too many things is certainly one of the major causes of psychic stress." He made a conscious effort to forget all that was not immediately important and committed all relevant data to paper "even at the price of having to prepare complex files." He claimed that this technique "can help anyone to accomplish the greatest simplicity compatible with the degree of complexity of his intellectual life." Sometimes stress arises from constantly postponing a particularly onerous or unpleasant job, which then hangs threateningly overhead like the sword of Damocles. This can be avoided by promoting this task to the top of the list so that it can be quickly dispatched and its threat removed.

- *Live a day at a time.* It is easy to be overawed by a work load spreading out for months ahead. Yet anyone is capable of coping with his allotted task for a period of twenty-four hours. Once that short span of work is completed it is equally easy to cope with the next day's load. Trouble arises when we permit our imaginations to dwell on the problems which we think will arise in the future. Then we suffer anticipatory stress. We must take the stand of Cardinal Newman who said: "I do not ask to see the distant scene, one step [is] enough for me"; or follow the advice of that wise nineteenth-century Canadian physician Sir William Osler, and "throw away all ambition beyond that of doing the day's work well."

- *Provide time for reflection.* The higher an executive climbs the less time he should spend in routine work, and the more time he should have free for quiet, creative thought. As Dr. H. Beric Wright, Medical Adviser to the British Institute of Directors, has said: "We would all benefit from more 'think time' in which to get things into better perspective." This particularly applies in times of crisis, when the tendency is to act first and regret afterward. One international airline company has erected a warning notice above the flight instrument panel of all their jets: "Before you do anything—do nothing." This cautionary note is aimed to prevent hasty, unconsidered action which has proved to be a common cause of pilot error, particularly among their junior staff. A similar custom applies in the British Royal Navy, where ships' captains, to prevent panic reaction in times of sudden disaster, give the order to "Sound the still." This is a call to crew members to stand calmly in their place for a few minutes before they start to follow their predetermined emergency drill.

- *Ensure sufficient variety of work.* The human body is so constructed that it never tires uniformly. As a result when we become fatigued, stressed, or inefficient in our performance of one particular task, we can often find renewal by switching to a different job. Variety of work is both the spice and savor of life. As Anatole France said, "Man is so made that he can only find relaxation from one labor by taking up another."

- *Enjoy your working life.* The man who derives enjoyment from his daily labors rarely suffers the effects of overwork however hard it may be. We suffer from a regime of "all work and no play" only because we need the relaxation of one to counterbalance the stimulus of the other. This was a point made by historian Edward Gibbon in *The History of the Decline and Fall of the Roman Empire.* Work, and the love of action, he said, "often leads to anger, to ambition and to revenge; but, when it is guided by the sense of propriety and benevolence, it becomes the parent of every virtue." This should be tempered by the love of pleasure so that, when "refined by art and learning, improved by the charms of social intercourse, and corrected by a just regard to economy, to health and to reputation, it is productive of the greatest part of the happines of private life." Ideally we should blend the Victorian work ethic with a hedonistic love of pleasure, for in Gibbon's words, "The character in which both the one and the other should be united and harmonized would seem to constitute the most perfect idea of human nature."

7
THE MARCH OF TIME

When a group of people were asked to select from a list of ten habits the factor which they believed to have contributed most to the heart attacks of their friends and business colleagues, seventy percent had no doubts in selecting "excessive competitive drive and meeting deadlines." In creating the clock we have created the instrument of our own destruction. Time we view as "the enemy" against which we are doomed to fight throughout our lives.

This antagonistic view of time received considerable reinforcement in Victorian England. "Every moment you now lose," Lord Chesterfield warned his readers, "is so much character and advantage lost, . . . every moment you now employ usefully, is so much time wisely laid out, at prodigious interest." Sloth and tardiness were naturally regarded as the cardinal sins in this era of unprecedented industrial growth. Even at the beginning of the eighteenth century, English factories employed monitors to record the comings and goings of the staff so that, in the words of the Law Book of the Crowley Iron Works, "sloth and villainy should be detected and the just and diligent rewarded." When the industrial time clock was introduced in 1895 it became possible to keep an automatic account of the time-keeping records of every employee and made it possible to dock fifteen minutes' wages from any worker who committed the unforgivable crime of arriving two minutes late for work, a practice still observed by some companies who continue to believe that hours of attendance are more important than either quality or quantity of work.

This approach to time is both damaging and unrealistic. We struggle to complete a task before the end of the working week, forgetting that the division of the year into fifty-two weeks is purely arbitrary. Now that we recognize nine planets orbiting around the sun we should, if we were logical, reorganize the year into weeks of ten days. This would have the immediate advantage of providing an additional seventy-two hours in each week's working schedule, enabling us to complete our appointed work with less haste. We really have the Benedictine monks to blame for our current obsession with time. It was they who pioneered the use of clocks in the Middle Ages. They created strict working timetables for themselves by dividing the period between sunrise and sunset into twelve daylight hours, each named after a devotional work. Prayers were alloted to them (Matins, Lauds, Prime, Terce, Sext, Nones, Vespers). Prior to this deadlines were unknown. Work was completed in the fullness of time, which could only be roughly measured by the burning of a candle, the shifting of a shadow on a sundial, or the movement of sand in an hourglass. It was only the invention of accurate chronometers that made it possible to keep appointments not simply "in the early forenoon" but at 8:15 precisely. It is this development more than anything else which has produced the hustle and bustle of contemporary Western life. Despite Einstein's revelations we continue to see time as a constantly flowing stream. People in the East are less inclined to fill the fleeting moments, for there emphasis is laid on the timeless "present." The Burmese, for example, have in their language no past or future tense. When they talk of events they do so with no reference to their time setting, and if they want to give an indication of the passage of time they do so in strictly practical terms, speaking of the period before sunset or the time it takes to cook a bowl of rice. For them time is not a commodity which can be made, had, saved or spent. Moreover since they hold to the karmic theory of life they have only a passing interest in punctuality. They believe that what is not done today or tomorrow can always be completed in the next life. We, on the other hand, are constantly struggling to maintain strict time schedules and herein lies an obvious and ubiquitous cause of stress.

When asked, many executives complained that the most potent source of strain in their work was the constant struggle to meet impossible deadlines. As was mentioned earlier, accountants, battling to complete their clients' financial returns before the end of the tax year, experience increasing strain and show a large rise in their blood-cholesterol level and a much more rapid clotting of their blood. Under this tension and with these biochemical changes they could easily suffer a heart attack. On the other hand, many creative workers find that they can only produce their best work when working against a strict deadline. This apparent paradox is explained by the Yerkes-Dodson law which, as explained previously, states that for the efficient performance of any task there is a certain optimum level of arousal. Exceed this level and we become less efficient, more anxious, and more prone to anxiety, fatigue and error. The awareness of time can therefore act as a spur or a scourge. It can drive us on to produce our finest work, or whip us into a state of nervous frenzy. Much depends on the reasonableness of the time schedule and the punishment for failure. If we try to read a library book the day before the last due date, we suffer little stress. We know that if we run short of time we can always skip the last chapter without anyone's finding out, or can take the book back a few days late and suffer no more than a token fine. But if failure to complete a task on time means we are likely to lose a large contract or forfeit our jobs, then we are likely to experience considerable stress.

Problems also arise when we try to perform more than one task at a time. This was an oft-recurring theme in our study of executive stress. A school principal complained that she was unable to get on with her work because of constant interruptions which broke her train of thought. A television producer believed his work would be relatively easy if he could concentrate on one task and not have to carry in his mind several shows all at various stages of development; and an advertising consultant said his major problem was the need to combine the different demands of creative work with the day-to-day chores of routine administration. The concurrence of conflicting work demands like these inevitably leads to stress. If we are to succeed in any endeavor we must be able to concentrate our attention and skills on the appointed task to the exclusion of everything else. As Ralph Waldo Emerson said, concentration is the "secret of strength in politics, in war, in trade—in short, in all the management of human affairs." When Lord Rosebery paid tribute to William Gladstone, the man many regard as having been England's most effective prime minister, he claimed that his greatest attribute "was his enormous power of concentration. There never was a man, I feel, in this world who, at any given moment, on any given subject, could so devote every resource and power of his intellect, without the restriction of a single nerve within him, to the immediate purpose of that subject." Those who can achieve this single-minded devotion are well on the way to securing their goal. Those whose attempts at concentration are thwarted are liable to suffer frustration and stress.

Of itself, concentration requires little effort. It is similar to the feat of burning a hole in a sheet of paper by concentrating the rays of sunlight through a magnifying glass. A powerful effect is obtained because all the available energy is focussed onto one particular spot. We laugh at inventors and lovers because of their supposed absent-mindedness, but they remain oblivious of the world around them not because they are absentminded, but because they are so absorbed in what they are doing that they lose awareness of everything else. Theirs is a state of total commitment, the enviable art of continuous and intense devotion to one particular cause. This is the secret of relaxed, powerful endeavor. Napoleon ascribed his success in battle to his ability to concentrate his forces on a single point in the enemy line. Writer Charles Kingsley also attributed his success to a talent for concentration. "I go at what I am about as if there were nothing else in the world for the time being. That's the secret of all hard-working men."

Time-linked stress can be minimized by adopting the following strategies:

- *Refuse to be obsessed with time.* The habit of constant clock-watching should be avoided, for it creates tension without generally improving performance. Recurrent shots of a clock relentlessly ticking away the minutes is a favorite device of moviemakers for creating tension as a film builds up to its final climax, but these *High Noon* tactics are pointless when applied in everyday life. Nervous glances at a watch will generate tension when you are caught in a cab in a traffic jam on the way to an important meeting, but they will not make the traffic move any faster. Punctuality may be the politeness of kings, but if your train is late, or your car is broken down, it may be impossible to keep an appointment on time. Fretting and fuming then will do nothing to rectify the situation. One needs to develop a more pragmatic approach to timekeeping. As the legendary Mayor Jimmy Walker of New York once said when criticized for arriving late for a public dinner: "If you're there before it's over, you're there on time." A clock is a most dangerous instrument to have in a car. We are not on racing circuits when we drive our cars and yet many people set themselves rigid lap times for the completion of their journeys. We can only travel at a certain maximum speed if we are to maintain a reasonable degree of safety, and that maximum speed depends to a very large extent on the prevailing road conditions. Since we have no control over the road conditions, we cannot expect to have absolute control over the time our trips take. Unfortunately this fact does not prevent our straining to cover the distance in a set time which, if we're even moderately competitive, will invariably be a few minutes quicker than our previous record time. This constant race with time leads to increased tension, fatigue and accidents, but precious little improvement in actual performance. As a test, two motorists were given the task of covering a distance of 1700 miles. One was asked to drive as fast as he could without breaking any speed limits, the other at a steady, comfortable pace. At the end of their journeys it was found that the fast driver had consumed ten gallons more gas and doubled the wear on his tires by driving at a speed which in the end proved to be only 2 m.p.h. faster than the other driver!

We should aim to imbue our lives with a little oriental calm. After all, the things we are doing now, and which seem so very important to us today, will probably be completely forgotten in a month or two. A useful test is to apply the advice given to Boswell by Dr. Johnson: "Sir, consider how insignificant this will appear a twelve-month hence." It takes a hundred years to create a mighty oak tree out of a tiny acorn, and no amount of forcing on our part will bring it to full maturity before its appointed time. We generally suffer needless frustration when we try to force the natural course of events, like the priest who grew increasingly irritated by the slow development of the work in his parish. Seeing his obvious agitation a visitor asked him what was wrong. "The trouble is," he replied, "that I'm in a hurry—but God isn't." Sometimes we need to learn the wisdom of letting things develop at their own pace and to follow the Taoist maxim: "Don't push the river, let it flow."

- *Work at your own pace.* As Shakespeare observed: "Time travels in divers pace with divers people."

With some it ambles, with others it trots. The wise man finds his own pace and sticks to it.

- *Plan the way you wish to apportion your time.* This advice was the essence of Arnold Bennett's best-selling book *How to Live on Twenty-four Hours a Day.* We all receive the same allotment of twenty-four hours per day and from this, as Bennett pointed out, "you have to spin health, pleasure, money, content, respect and the evolution of your immortal soul." We stand little chance of achieving any of these goals unless we establish a definite plan for the use of our time. Unless we establish control over the way we use our time we must find, as Seneca said, "There are some hours which are taken from us, some which are stolen from us, and some which slip from us." Many businessmen say that if only they had the time they would like to study a foreign language, but what they really mean is that on Thursday when they could be attending an evening class in Spanish they prefer to watch television. Others say that given the time they would like to read the works of the world's great philosophers. If they spent less time reading the repetitive, ephemeral news in the daily papers they would have ample time in the course of a year to read several major philosophical works. It is a question of personal choice and disciplined application; we must set realistic goals and then work steadily toward their achievement. It is no good adopting the task of writing a book unless we also set aside the necessary time for carrying out the work. Since getting started is half the battle, it is also necessary to establish definite starting dates.

50
129

Footprints in the sands of time are never made by sitting down. When we are given a work load which obviously exceeds the time available for its completion we must either argue in advance for a later completion date, be prepared to delegate some of the work or be willing to accept a lower standard of work.

- *Provide definite breathing spaces during the day's schedule.* Many people if they have a spare hour during the day will automatically try to fill it with an appointment or visit. Work, following Parkinson's Law and nature's abhorrence of a vacuum, has an unhappy knack of expanding to fill the time available. Most people choose to keep their appointment books overfilled. To curb this unfortunate tendency, try to plan breaks to be used if all goes well as "thinking time," but which can, if necessary, be used to complete work which has been unavoidably delayed. This avoids the stressful situation of being behind schedule and constantly struggling to catch up.

- *Keep the schedules flexible.* We should be prepared to work a longer or shorter working day as the occasion demands. The introduction of *gleitende arbeitszeit* (staggered work time) in Germany has resulted in increased production and a reported decrease in absenteeism.

- *Live a day a time.* Sir William Osler, a former Regius Professor of Medicine at Oxford University, told a meeting of students that the secret of his success was that he had learned to live his life "in day-tight compartments." Anyone can carry his load of trouble until nightfall. We inflict unnecessary strain when we concern ourselves with the failures of the past and the projected disasters of the future as well as the problems of the present. As the revised standard version of St. Matthew's Gospel puts it, "Be not anxious for tomorrow, for tomorrow will be anxious for itself. Let the day's own troubles be sufficient for the day."

- *Cultivate the habit of concentration.* Concentration is an art which is rarely practiced today. We discourage people from developing their minds by providing them with rapidly changing TV shows, short news flashes, book digests and picture-filled tabloid newspapers. So it becomes second nature to pick up a book, read a few pages and then skip to the end; to take an adult education course, study the first few lessons and then lose interest; or start a business venture and then quit when it is just about to get off the ground. The habit of steady application can be acquired by making a point of concentrating fully on every task we undertake, whether it is working, reading, playing cards, or listening to stereo records.

  Time-wasting, stress-producing interruptions must also be reduced. Research at Cambridge University has shown that senior executives often spend only one-fifth of their time on creative work, with the remainder wasted on interruptions and breakdowns in the system of internal communication. These interruptions can be reduced by delegating more, by encouraging subordinates to work without constant referral and by training secretaries to be more effective guardians of their bosses' time

8

THE STRUGGLE FOR STATUS

When we assess strangers, one of the first questions we ask is "What do they do?" Newspapers will report a collision involving not a man and a woman, but a forty-six-year-old sales executive and his forty-four-year-old wife. We feel we know something about the characters involved the moment we know the work they do.

In primitive times a man was sometimes judged by his possessions, by the size of his flock of sheep or the extent of his land. More often his renown rested on his personal attributes as expressed in feats of wisdom, skill and daring. Solomon is remembered today more for his store of wisdom than for the size of his harem; King Arthur for his chivalrous acts; Joan of Arc for her courage; the Black Prince for his skill in battle and Robin Hood for his relentless fight against oppression and social injustice. The most cherished quality an Anglo-Saxon could possess was *lof*, a term which is difficult to translate accurately but which roughly means the praise and esteem of his fellows. The term recurs frequently in *Beowulf*, the eighth-century epic poem, which tells how Beowulf delivered the Danish King Brothgar from the water-demon Grendel and so won the plaudits of his kinsmen and the epitaph "the gentlest of men, the kindest to his people and the most desirous of *lof*."

Fame today cannot be achieved this way. There are now no water-demons left to kill, no fiery dragons for St. George to slay, and no maidens to be rescued from ivory towers or Minoan labyrinths. The modern Galahad, if he wants to seek public acclaim, is more likely to find it in the boardroom than on the battlefield. In today's society it is mainly through our work that we achieve status, identity and personal validation. This explains the importance of the rat race and the constant competitive struggle for supremacy, which psychologist Alfred Adler saw as one of our primary sources of motivation. Moving for the first time into a private office with wall-to-wall carpeting and an antique desk can be a source of deep satisfaction. Equally well, a demotion, even if it means no more than losing access to the executive dining room, can be the cause of considerable distress. As Norman O. Brown writes: "The need of the individual for status and function is the most significant of his traits, and if this need remains unsatisfied nothing else can compensate for its lack." The provision of status is an essential part of job enrichment, and the loss of status a major problem at times of retirement or unemployment. Lord Beveridge was convinced that the greatest evil of unemployment was not poverty, but that it makes men "seem useless, not wanted." Even the most generous social benefits cannot fill this need. Unemployment and under-employment have a disastrous effect on the national economy, but the loss is small compared with the psychological damage done to the individuals themselves. Studies have shown that the unemployed worker loses self-confidence and rapidly develops feelings of worthlessness and inferiority. Similar changes are seen in people who on reaching retirement age suddenly find themselves abandoned, put out to grass to while away their remaining days.

Unfortunately, while it was simple for a skilled craftsman to derive a sense of satisfaction and personal achievement from his work, this is far less easy for the modern factory or office worker. Even the executive stands so far removed from the end point of his labors that he frequently finds it difficult to assess the value of his individual work. There is little that is distinctive about the contribution he makes, and he knows that he could be easily replaced. Any feedback he gets from his "customers" is more likely to be critical than supportive. So he comes to feel alienated, unfulfilled and ultimately resentful of a system which deprives him of a basic source of satisfaction. As psychiatrist Anthony Storr writes, "When a man is, or feels himself to be, an unimportant cog in a very large machine, he is deprived of the chance of aggressive self-affirmation, and a proper pride and dignity." This, he believes, arouses early childhood feelings of weakness and helplessness with a corresponding tendency for his unexpressed, normal aggression to turn into hate and resentment. Interpersonal stress in industry can often be traced back to the conflicts, disappointments, frustrations and harbored resentments involved in the constant struggle to achieve supremacy.

It is wrong, however, to regard the struggle for status as purely negative in its effect. Ethological studies have shown that the stability of animal communities depends on the establishment of a clearly defined hierarchy. The early work of the Norwegian Schjelderup-Ebbe showed that a flock of hens rapidly organizes itself into a clearly demarcated "pecking order," in which the dominant bird has the right to peck all others without the risk of being pecked in return. The middle of the ranking order is organized rather like a ladder, with birds free to do battle only with those directly above or below them in the hierarchy. This strict ranking system, although maintained by force, helps to achieve peace by reducing the amount of conflict within a group. Observations show that once a well-defined pecking order has been established within a flock of chickens, the birds are less aggressive, eat more heartily, maintain a better weight and lay more eggs. Tension arises only when the social structure of the flock is upset, for instance by the arrival of alien birds.

The creation of a definite hierarchy is even more important among the larger primates, which depend for their survival when attacked, not on a disorderly retreat into the trees, but on concerted defense. The ceaseless struggle for supremacy is vital for baboons, for example, for it ensures that the troop is led by the strongest member. Under him will be a disciplined ranking order, which reduces internal conflicts and enables controlled defensive action to be taken when the troop is attacked from outside. In order to make this endless quest worthwhile, Nature has provided rewards for animals who climb the pecking order, and penalities for those who fall. Those who climb become elated, which helps increase their dominance. Those who fall become dejected, depressed and apathetic, which strips them of their desire to fight back, and makes it easier for them to accept their lowered status. As Humphrey Knipe and George Maclay point out in their study of *The Dominant Man*, "Whatever the form of the competition—whether the rivalries of the stock market or a contest for political leadership—the emotional consequences of winning and losing remain the same. The winner experiences an immediate rise in ego level, a thrill of elation which he inevitably communicates to others through an increase in assertiveness and self-confidence. The loser is overcome with despondency. His social behavior becomes more than usually inhibited and he may withdraw altogether from social relationships." Violent mood swings can occur if these hierarchical movements are excessively rapid, as when a national leader is catapulted to a position of totalitarian control and shows signs of megalomaniacal elation, or when a deposed President on his fall from grace sinks into a state of deep depression and suicidal despair. In many ways the struggle for supremacy within human groups has outlived its survival value, and one can frequently notice unfortunate outcomes of our continuing pursuance of this atavistic hierarchical struggle.

In certain companies it produces a level of competition which is harmful to the individual and damaging to the long-term interests of the group. It ensures that ambitious individuals, in accordance with the Peter Principle, rise in the hierarchy until they reach the level of their own incompetence. Here they remain firmly supported by their reputation and track record, for there appears to be no need for dominant *Homo sapiens* to be constantly proving their worth as is necessary in other animal hierarchies. Many managers rise up the managerial hierarchy on spurious grounds and for reasons which may not make them suitable for corporate leadership. To promote an electronics engineer to a position of senior management simply because of his technical expertise is to mistake his value to the group. He may be good at programming computers but hopeless at handling men. The same applies to military commanders. Dr. Norman Dixon, Reader in

Psychology at University College, London, has made a special study of the psychology of military incompetence. He finds that junior officers are promoted for qualities of conformity and obedience which do not fit them for ultimate control. Problems arise, he points out, "when such a person reaches a position of top command because this type of personality—over-controlled, obsessive, dogmatic, authoritarian, and having a 'close mind'—is ill-tuned to the job of high-level decision-making. Such people are intolerant of ambiguity and uncertainty, they are inflexible, unimaginative, unrealistic in their risk-taking and inclined to remember and perceive only those things which are palatable and do not arouse anxiety."

Further problems arise because the human drive to achieve dominance is not motivated by a simple striving after excellence, but by a host of other complex and often conflicting forces. Dr. Pierre Rentchnik, a Swiss medical researcher, studied the lives of over three hundred political and religious leaders and found that a remarkably high percentage of them—including Lloyd George, Ivan the Terrible, Attila, Ataturk, Lenin, Stalin, Hitler and Hadrian—were either orphaned or lost their fathers at an early age. Others—Calvin, Churchill, Martin Luther, Mao Tse-tung, Nasser, President Tito, Golda Meir and ex-President Nixon—were, as children, rejected or abandoned by their fathers. As a result, he concluded: "The orphan in search of security becomes aggressive and tries to dominate society and destiny." A similar study showed that sixty-seven percent of British prime ministers from Walpole to Chamberlain had suffered the loss of a parent in childhood or early adolescence, which, in the opinion of researcher Lucille Iremonger, explained both their subsequent drive for power and the frequently noted contrast between their outward show of gregariousness and geniality with "the intense sensitivity, isolation and solitariness of their true natures."

A similar conflict is noticeable in the personalities of many successful businessmen who conceal behind a façade of extroversion the temperament of a born loner. In other instances the overwhelming drive to achieve dominance appears to stem from early feelings of inferiority. This was probably so in the case of Napoleon, who created an empire and married an aristocrat to help compensate for his puny stature and humble birth. Similarly with the immigrant Jews who overcame their feelings of rootlessness and financial insecurity by traveling to America where they proceeded to amass fortunes and to found dynasties of worldwide renown.

You do not have to be neurotic to succeed in business, but it certainly seems to help. The tendency is, as J. F. Nisbet concluded in his study *The Insanity of Genius*, "the greater the genius, the greater the unsoundness." This provides the necessary driving force as we strive for compensatory attention, adulation and success. But there is room for only one leader at the head of every pack, and as firms get larger there will be fewer opportunities for the man of naturally high dominance to achieve a position of ultimate power. This must inevitably increase the competitive struggle to reach the top, and the dissatisfaction experienced lower down the hierarchy. With fewer pools it will be less easy to be a big fish in a small pond, and an increasing number of executives will have to be content to be small fry in a large organization.

Fortunately there are several ways to lessen the stressful impact of the human hierarchical struggle:

- *Establish stable hierarchies.* Organizations must endeavor to establish stable hierarchies, for humans as well as chickens are happier and function more effectively in a stable social environment. In times of social unrest mental illness increases. It falls in communities where there is a strict caste system in which everyone knows his or her role and place. The stability of a group can be increased by providing a strong leader who discourages squabbling among subordinates; by the creation of ranking laws, orders of precedence, titles and hierarchical perquisites; and by aggressive involvement with rival groups. All these techniques can be usefully employed in industry to avoid internecine strife.

- *Honest self-appraisal.* Individuals must strive for a more realistic appraisal of their own abilities and needs. It is better to join the right company and climb slowly to the top than join the "big boys" of a major corporation and suffer a series of humiliating defeats. We unquestionably accept that every private should strive to attain the rank of general, but does everybody really want to be a leader? After all, why struggle to climb the pecking order if you feel the rewards are only chicken feed?

  Most people show a discrepancy between their public image, self-image and ego-ideal (the sort of person they would like to become). They suffer stress and loss of self-esteem only when the gap between these concepts grows too great and reality as they perceive it bears no relation to either their hopes or public façade. This happens, for example, when a fading movie star finds it increasingly difficult to live up to her public image as a beautiful sex goddess. This common source of stress can be alleviated by making an honest self-appraisal and then either modifying our goals, presenting a more honest public front or by endeavoring by a steady process of self-improvement to more nearly reach our ego-ideal.

- *Flexible role playing.* We must achieve greater flexibility in the roles we play. Everyone at some time in his life has to play both dominant and submissive roles. During the week a man may be a highly respected senior executive in the office, a choir member in the church, a struggling novice on the golf course and a general drudge in the home. The word "person" derives from the Latin *persona,* meaning a player's mask or the character in a play. Our personalities represent the sum total of the roles we choose to play on the stage of life. The successful person, like a competent repertory actor, has the confidence and ability to move easily from role to role. This makes him more colorful and more adept at handling a variety of situations.

- *Generous use of public approval and praise.* The estimate we make of our status and worth depends to a very large extent on the feedback we get from our colleagues. Praise increases our self-esteem, while blame heightens our sense of failure and inferiority. A number of studies have been made of the effects of praise and reprimand on the quality and quantity of work performed by students. These show that the finest incentive is public praise which improves performance in 87.5 percent of cases. Other incentives in descending order of effectiveness are private reprimand, public reprimand, private ridicule, public ridicule and private sarcasm. At the bottom of the list is public sarcasm, which in

65.1 percent of cases results in a deterioration of performance. Approval raises morale and gains a cooperative response, whereas criticism begets sullen resistance. Far more could be done in news releases to the local press to praise the work of individual employees, and corporate advertisements should be used not only to plug the firm's products but also to praise the technical abilities of its staff. Company newsletters should also make a point of mentioning achievements of employees as well as their ability to retire, change departments, produce children, get married, engaged or die.

- *Prepare the way for your promotion.* It is easier for a group to accept the elevation in status of one of its members if the individual temporarily quits the group and then returns. This is a strategy commonly employed by native tribes and described by Martin Page in *The Company Savage* as "ritual absence." Both Mohammed and Christ spent a period of isolation in the mountains before they returned to join their people. This made it easier for them to be accepted in their new roles. Newlyweds go away on a honeymoon, and are then welcomed back by their families as a full-fledged married couple. In the same way, politicians embark on world tours to enhance their status at home, and concert pianists go abroad to advance their reputation with their fellow countrymen. A ritual absence can also benefit executives faced with promotion above their peers. Taking a three-month course, accepting temporary assignment to another company or taking substantial leave to carry out research will help to ease the hierarchical transition and reduce intragroup tension.

9
DECISION-MAKING

A manager exists to make decisions. A large part of his skill lies in his ability to choose between alternative courses of action, each of which must be carefully evaluated according to its rival merits. What markets should be entered? What range of products manufactured? What staff employed? What finance raised? Sometimes these decisions are easily made. More often they are exceedingly complex and involve a host of variables and an irreducible handful of unknown factors. Stress arises if we are unable to choose between the various possible courses of action, and substitute inaction and indecision for decisive purposeful action. On these occasions we may rationalize our conduct by saving we choose to "play it by ear," or are content to "wait and see which way the wind blows." But whether we recognize it or not we generally suffer anxiety when we remain helpless pawns in the hand of fate. California psychologists Peter Lindsay and Donald Norman, in their wide-ranging study of the decision-making process, recognize the frequency of this plight. "It is no wonder that the sheer complexity of reaching a decision often causes one to give up in despair, postponing the event for as long as possible, sometimes actually making the final choice only when forced, and then often without any attempt to consider all the implications of that choice."

As society grows increasingly complex so do the problems of executive decision-making. Problems arise in industry where a selection has to be made between machinery and processes which may appear to have identical merits. Even if the choice can be narrowed down to two competing machines how can one feel any great assurance in deciding between a machine which is ten percent neater than its rival, twenty percent safer, fifteen percent more reliable, eight percent cheaper, but twenty-eight percent slower? Added to this are the problems of uncertainty. How can one be sure that a technical breakthrough will not make both machines obsolete within the next two years? Is there any certainty that the demand for the product will continue long enough to justify the capital output? Equally important, will the government continue to make generous allowances for plant depreciation or will changes in tax laws and a sudden increase in interest rates make it more attractive to rent rather than make an outright purchase of the machine? Uncertainties like these create anxiety by making clear-cut decisions difficult if not impossible.

Laboratory experiments have shown that animals do not like uncertainty. Groups of rats were given the opportunity of following two maze pathways at the ends of which there might or might not be a food reward. One pathway was provided with clear markings which indicated whether or not there would be food at the end of the maze, the other carried no such clues. Though the marking made no difference to the end result, it was found that the rats showed a marked preference for the maze which eliminated all uncertainty and let them know in advance what lay in store for them. Experience suggests that the same applies to human behavior. When given the chance we too prefer to know what lies ahead, even if that knowledge cannot affect the outcome of events.

Errors invariably creep into the decision-making process when we cannot eliminate the element of chance. For one thing, we tend to overestimate the occurrence of events with high probability. Similarly we are prone to overestimate the likelihood of events we want to happen, and underestimate those we hope will not occur. The wise manager, faced with uncertainty, learns to eliminate these common biases from his reckoning.

In addition to the growing complexity of choice and the increasing uncertainty of modern business life, the executive is also in the invidious position of being rarely able to act either spontaneously or intuitively. Before he acts he must always go through the often agonizing process of weighing up the pros and cons. The options open to Stone Age man were few and quickly resolved. If he came face-to-face with a saber-toothed tiger he had little alternative but to stand his ground and fight, or take to his legs and flee. Survival in the contemporary jungle is infinitely more complex. With our highly developed intellect and strong powers of imagination we can see ranging in front of us an infinite number of alternative courses of action, each with its individual ramifications and envisaged consequences. Decision-making under these circumstances becomes a source of so much anxiety that we frequently balk at the task rather than run the risk of making a wrong choice. As Sir Heneage Ogilvie concluded, "A prominent component of stress is indecision, and a factor in anti-stress is undoubtedly the power of decision." If we are to remain serene we need to solve outstanding problems, resolve conflict and, as far as possible, banish uncertainty. This is the art of effective executive control. Unfortunately the process of managerial selection does not always take this faculty into account. Managers are frequently appointed, not because they have the ability to make sound decisions, but because they are intelligent, personable or technically proficient.

This happens when an able administrator is promoted to a position where he has to initiate action as well as carry it out. Such people are often inflexible, unimaginative, intolerant of uncertainty and unwilling to risk any great departure from the tried and tested routines. These qualities may make for success in an office manager, but are likely to prove a disaster in a marketing director. It should never be assumed that an efficient second-in-command will necessarily make an adequate boss. The job requirements may be totally different. Unfortunately this is rarely discovered until the promotion is made. All too often the Peter Principle operates and a man is consistently promoted until he reaches the level of his own, often patently obvious, incompetence.

Our ability to make effective decisions is subject to considerable variation. Some individuals find the strain intolerable, like the grocer's assistant who attributed his nervous breakdown to a minor promotion, which meant he had to assume the responsibility for grading oranges according to size, sorting the large from the small. This had caused him great anxiety. "The whole day it's decisions, decisions, decisions," he told a hospital psychiatrist. At the other end of the scale are the men who can, without batting an eyelid, make policy decisions involving themselves or their firms in an outlay of millions of dollars.

Fortunately much can be done to improve the effectiveness, and reduce the strain, of executive decision-making:

- *Avoid unnecessary problems.* "The buck stops here" was the famous note on President Truman's desk, but often the buck should not have got there in the first place. Senior management should keep their probing fingers out of petty office problems. Let the personnel department decide whether to transfer a filing clerk because she is at loggerheads with the office manager, or having an affair with the sales director.

- *Tackle decision-making in an orderly fashion.* Before making a final decision on any subject, whether it is the problem of how to allocate a firm's capital resources, what shares of stock to hold in a private portfolio or where to go for a vacation, it pays to follow four basic steps:

  1. Make a detailed statement of the problem.
  2. Formulate all possible solutions.
  3. Evaluate the possible alternatives.
  4. Select the best solution.

  This is the policy advocated for infantry officers who are trained to make a careful appreciation of every military situation. This follows a standard drill: a statement of the aim; a review of possible courses of action; a selection of the best course; and finally, the formulation of a detailed plan. Experience has shown that following this painstaking routine helps to prevent hasty, ill-considered action.

- *Set clear goals.* Problems can be broken down into two main categories—well-defined problems and ill-defined problems. The difference between them lies simply in the clarity of the goal. We get good answers only when we ask the right questions. Maybe the sales of one particular product are slumping badly despite an intensive television advertising campaign, and the question asked is "How can we stimulate sales?" As a result a host of decisions are made to alter the packaging, decrease the price, introduce a special premium offer and change to a different advertising agency. But still sales fall. Possibly the answers were sound, but maybe the question itself was at fault. Perhaps the initial query should have been "Is there a demand for this particular product at this particular time?" Too often operational decisions are taken, while strategic problems themselves are ignored.

Frequently a network of sub-goals has to be established in addition to the central goal. The overriding principle of most executive decisions is to maximize corporate gains, but the maximum return on capital invested does not necessarily represent the maximum long-term gain for either the company, its employees, stockholders or society at large. Often it may also be necessary to aim to maximize minimum gains and minimize maximum losses. Sub-goals such as these need to be clearly stated if orderly decisions are to be made.

- *Commit as much as possible to writing.* A pen and pencil can be the decision-maker's greatest aids. Stress arises when our mental computers are overloaded with a mass of unprocessed, uncoordinated data. However great or little our intellectual ability we all share the same limited short-term memory.

At any time we can carry in our minds a maximum of only about seven units of information. As a result, while we can comfortably carry out the mental multiplication of 72 x 8, we find it exceedingly difficult to do the same with the figures 72 x 38 because this requires us to carry ten figures in our mind, a load which exceeds our short-term memory capacity. This is where a calculator or a sheet of paper becomes helpful.

The use of pen and paper also helps us follow the decision-making process in an orderly fashion and to keep track while doing so of any number of sub-goals. Many of the problems an executive has to solve are similar to the hardy perennial "If the puzzle you solved before you solved this one was harder than the puzzle you solved after you solved the puzzle before you solved this one, was the puzzle you solved before you solved this one harder than this one?" A mind-boggling task, unless carried out systematically with pencil and paper.

- *Obtain the maximum possible information* relevant to the task. This can be done by study, by sounding out the opinions of business colleagues and friends or by holding "brainstorming" sessions when a group of six or more people get together to produce as many solutions as possible to the one particular problem. The important thing with these sessions is to suspend all ridicule and criticism, for even the most far-fetched idea can be the starting point of a brilliant creative innovation.

Sometimes in order to ensure a sufficiently comprehensive gathering of information it pays to follow a routine system of inquiry. Medical students are trained to take a case history by first asking the patient for details of their age, occupation, personal history, habits and personal health record. This helps to ensure that no vital data are ignored before an attempt is made to formulate a diagnosis. In the same way one team of mechanical engineers has found it easier to solve their particular technical problems if they go through the routine of finding answers to queries: Other ruses? Borrow or adapt? New twist? More so? Less so? Substitutes? Rearrange? Reverse? Combine?

The important thing is to avoid the tendency to think along limited stereotyped lines. Do not be content until you have turned the problem upsidedown and viewed it from all possible angles. Scores of people tried to find an orthodox solution to the problems presented by a truck stuck fast under a low bridge, before a youngster came along and suggested they should deflate the truck's tires. Dr. Edward de Bono, director of the Cognitive Research Trust at Cambridge, gives a further example of this process which he describes as "lateral thinking." An ambulance rushing along a country road suddenly confronts a herd of sheep blocking its way. The natural reaction is for the driver to pick his way slowly through the flock. A more effective response, apparent immediately to anyone trained in the process of lateral thinking, is to stop the ambulance and drive the flock past the stationary vehicle.

- *Gain experience in decision-making*, for the more experience we have the fewer mistakes we make and the less anxiety we suffer. The corporate whiz kid may be able to offer initiative, drive and youth-ful exuberance, but if he lacks experience, he lacks one of the essential ingredients for successful executive decision-making. In a game of chess the possible permutations for a sequence of eight con-secutive moves run to over a million billion billion. No chess master could hope to evaluate all these combinations. His skill lies in the ability, gained through long experience, of recognizing certain patterns of play and mastering certain basic strate-gies. Throughout the game he chooses moves which give his opponent the minimum number of replies, and help him to control the center of the board. In managing the end play he gives priority to checks which add a new piece to the attack, which use the most powerful possible piece, or which offer him a double check (when his opponent's king is threatened by two or more pieces). In this way he simplifies the game and reduces the number of moves he has to consider and evaluate. The prac-ticed executive handles his business decisions in a similar way. He recognizes from past experience certain common themes and underlying chords which simplify his choice and reduce the uncer-tainty of his action, and add confidence to his judg-ment.

- *Avoid undue procrastination.* When there is no pressure to make a snap decision it may occasionally help to set the problem to one side and come back to it at a later date when fresh information is avail-able, or when the mysterious workings of the un-conscious mind have had a chance to produce an unmeditated solution. But more often than not procrastination of this kind merely lengthens the period of stressful indecision and ensures that when a decision is finally made it is made in haste and under duress. Louis Halle is convinced that this is a common failure of contemporary politicians. "One of the reasons for the rarity of statesmanship is that, in a world increasingly rushed to death, the long range waits on the immediate. What is urgent takes priority over what is merely important, so that what is important will be attended to only when it becomes urgent, which may be too late."

In order to avoid the dangers of indecisive floundering, infantry officers are trained to take firm courageous action even at the risk of making the occasional mistake. "To do the right thing is commendable," they are told; "to do the wrong thing is regrettable; to do nothing is unforgivable." This is the maxim which could be followed with profit by vacillating executives. You cannot win them all, but if you do not take a chance, you will not win any of them. When in doubt it is often better to make up your mind by the toss of a coin than make no decision at all. That way you at least avoid the strain of constant indecision.

- *Avoid post-mortems* and post-decisional recriminations. Learn from your mistakes, but never allow them to become a source of constant self-reproach. Follow the practice of Abraham Lincoln who, when carrying the enormous responsibilities of the Civil War, made the decisions he felt to be right irrespective of the criticism they might incur. As he said, "If the end brings me out right, what is said against me won't amount to anything. If the end brings me out wrong, ten angels swearing I was right would make no difference."

10
THE MARCH TOWARD AUTONOMY

Work provides us with an opportunity to satisfy many of our basic needs. Even the most humble job provides an income which can be used to buy the basic essentials for survival—food, clothing and shelter. Less mundane tasks also afford a chance of self-expression and emotional release. Professor Scott Myers, who worked as a psychologist at the Texas Instruments Co., divides these needs into two main categories: "Maintenance" needs (pay, physical conditions of working environment, security, status) and "motivational" needs (possibility of growth, achievement, recognition and responsibility). In the past both management and unions have concentrated on satisfying the "maintenance" needs of workers. Now that these basic physical needs are being more adequately met, industry must advance to giving far greater consideration to the satisfaction of the less tangible but nonetheless potent "motivation" needs.

Abraham Maslow, a leading exponent of the school of humanistic psychology, showed that each one of us has a hierarchy of needs, arranged in ascending order from the most primitive animal needs to the highest cultural aspirations. At the base level lies the instinctive drive to satisfy our craving for food, drink and sex. Once these basic physiological needs have been met we progress to seeking security. Then, once our safety has been assured, we climb a further rung of the ladder of desire and seek the love and company of our fellow beings. When this has been secured we take a further step and try to achieve self-esteem, and later still self-fulfillment. Each time we set our sights a little higher and aim to satisfy a higher level of need. A Bantu tribesman may spend a large part of his time hunting game, but the need of the executive is not for food, of which he generally has far too much, but for self-assertion. As Laurie Taylor, Professor of Sociology at the University of York, has said, "The construction of an identity is the single most important problem for contemporary individuals, once beyond food, housing and some sort of security." When we are thwarted in our quest to establish a strong sense of personal identity we will, Professor Taylor finds, use vacations, hobbies, sex, drugs or even magic in an attempt to assert that "I am not like all those other people, this is the real me." Unfortunately, it is becoming increasingly difficult to assert our individuality in a world of growing conformity, complexity and size.

In primitive communities action was rewarded and worry punished. The man who fought off a marauding bear survived, the man who sat down and worried about what to do next inevitably perished. Today the position is often reversed and society punishes the man of action whose conduct offends in any way its myriad rules and regulations, and rewards instead the man who remains inert for fear of breaking even the smallest point of the law. This gives rise to the professional automatons found in all large firms, the men who always obey but never decide, whose only creative action is to formulate new laws or tighten up the enforcement of existing regulations. For them the means are always more important than the ends.

If we are to stimulate creativity in industry we must give individuals more freedom to develop and express their own ideas. As William Whyte observed: "People very rarely *think* in groups; they talk together, they exchange information, they adjudicate, they make compromises. But they do not think; they do not create." If a revolutionary idea is put to a committee it will rarely be greeted with support. Committees are always more conservative than individuals. Their survival depends on a consensus of opinion, and this is rarely gained for a very simple reason. The harmony of a group is jealously guarded by its members, and since a new idea must of necessity challenge existing practice and disturb the status quo, the group will invariably shelve the idea rather than risk disrupting the harmony of the team. At the same time they will make suitable placatory noises to the scheme's proponent who is then forced to conceal his frustration and swallow his pride until he can hassle, lobby, cajole and flatter sufficiently to get the scheme adopted. This is a common cause of stress among executives, who know their ideas are sound, but cannot get them accepted by those in a position of power.

When questioned about the major sources of stress in their working lives many executives complained of the frustration of constant bureaucratic interference. An administrative nurse complained that she could not get on with running her hospital because of the need for constant reference to the regional hospital board, to whom she had to make endless accounts of staff attendance, sickness records and patients' complaints. An architect said his work would be relatively pleasant except for the constant battle with local planning authorities over every petty building regulation.

This is a source of friction throughout the world. In Sweden, anyone wanting to build a house to his own design rather than purchase a standard model has to fill in 192 forms. In France it is estimated that even small companies employing less than ten in staff have to spend thirty-five hours a month filling in government forms—one of which inquires how much water leaves the work place seventy-five percent dirty, fifty percent dirty and twenty-five percent dirty! The virtual impossibility of making this assessment with any degree of accuracy makes no difference to the fine which is extracted for noncompletion of the form. In England successive chancellors have befuddled the electorate with a bewildering array of new tax laws from CGT and SET, VAT, DGT, DLT, PRT, and CTT. In America, according to a recent poll, two-thirds of the population regret the increasing tendency of government to impinge upon their daily lives.

James H. Boren, head of an engineering and design firm, now spends a large part of his time lecturing and writing books aimed at the inefficiencies of the U.S. bureaucratic machine. He sees their contribution to the commercial scene as one of "dynamic inaction, decision-postponement patterns and creative status quo." They "fuzzify" everything, he claims, to permit an "adjustive interpretation" at a later date, and constantly postpone decisions in the hope that they will either disappear or land on someone else's desk.

Somehow the individual has to fight to exert his autonomy in a world of impersonal, megalithic corporations and increasingly totalitarian governments. Junior executives must insist on the introduction of "participation management," for only when they are brought into the decision-making process will they escape frustration and be able to relate their personal goals to that of the company for which they work. Senior executives must see that their jobs are modified to make full use of their talents and creative skill, rather than submit, like Procrustes, to manipulations which tailor them to fit arbitrarily limited job specifications. At the end of a working lifetime we should be able to say that, right or wrong, "I did it my way." We will then become the sort of people described by Abraham Maslow as "self-actualising people," by psychoanalyst Carl Jung as "individuated people," and by philosopher Eric Fromm as "autonomous people."

These are mature people who are so sure of their own identity, and possess so high a degree of self-acceptance, that they do not need to hide their faults or pretend to be what they are not. These are the people who are content to make up their own minds about the quality of a wine without first reading the label, independent individuals who can tolerate uncertainty without feeling threatened, and who are not afraid to admit their ignorance when floundering in the dark. These are the people who can exercise managerial control with minimum stress. Yes-men are useless in the higher echelons of business. Industry needs at its helm rugged individualists who are prepared to steer by the seat of their pants, not by a standard manual of seamanship. If faceless automatons do get into the boardroom occasionally, it is likely that they will do so, in the words of J. Paul Getty, "only to set out the writing pads or empty the ashtrays."

The firm that has the courage to grant its executives greater autonomy will enjoy increased production and far greater job satisfaction. The American Telephone and Telegraph Company found there was a high degree of discontent among the women working in the difficult departments of consumer relations. A business management consultant called in to investigate the problem found that the employees—seventy percent of whom were highly skilled college graduates—were dissatisfied because their work was being subjected to excessive scrutiny from above. Job satisfaction soared when they were encouraged to become experts in the problems which really interested them, and allowed to work with minimum supervision. "All we did, really," said a personnel executive, "was to let them make more and more decisions about their work as they became experienced." As a result staff turnover dropped, job satisfaction increased and the number of complaints received from customers plummeted.

The higher the level of managerial responsibility the greater the need for autonomy, and the greater the frustration experienced when this freedom of individual action is curtailed. A comparative study of top managers and those at a lower level showed that top managers did not rate themselves particularly highly on intelligence and were not highly motivated to seek power, job security or financial reward. They saw as their main attribute the ability to take the initiative, and their major driving force the need for achievement, self-expression and personal fulfillment. "They are pioneers rather than consolidators, and are seeking fulfillment through achievement rather than rewards or security," said Professor C. K. Elliott, Professor of Human Resources Management at England's Loughborough University.

Executives suffer stress when this striving for self-assertion is blocked. This can be avoided by the following strategies:

- *Adopt a policy of quiet but firm self-assertion.* Sometimes a showdown or aggressive face-to-face confrontation is necessary to defend one's autonomy or personal integrity. Like a surgical operation it can be painful at the time, but may in the long run be the only way of obtaining permanent relief from an intolerable situation.

As politicians have frequently discovered, a secure peace is rarely achieved by a policy of constant compromise and appeasement. A boss does not earn the freedom to be independent and idiosyncratic as a result of attaining a position of senior managerial control; it is through the exercise of independent thought and action that he proves himself worthy of becoming the boss.

Similarly we must not allow ourselves to be unduly influenced by the criticisms or hostility of others. To be fully mature we must overcome unnecessary and limiting dependency patterns and come to rely more and more on our own ideas, opinions and judgment. As American lawyer John Foster has said, "One of the strongest characteristics of genius is the power of lighting its own fire." The successful manager lights his own fire and pursues his objectives without fear of failure or criticism. He follows in his life the epitaph inscribed on the grave of the Cretan writer Nikos Kazantzakis, author of *Zorba the Greek*: "I fear nothing. I hope for nothing. I am free."

- *Avoid jobs which limit autonomy and growth.* Many firms attempt to disprove the old saying: "You can't keep a good man down." They fail only because the good man refuses to stay in a dead job where there is insufficient scope for the full exercise of his talents and skills. This in fact is the major cause of job transfer among executives. One well-known firm of management consultants asked 422 job-hunting executives why they were seeking a move. They found that the main reason was to find a job which offered more scope, more responsibility and more challenge. As William Lear, founder of Lear Inc., says, "As soon as you've learned how to do your job as well as it can be done, ask for more responsibility in your company—or for a different job. If you don't get it, get the hell out!" Alternatively go solo, even if to begin with it means more responsibility and a greatly reduced income.

- *Broaden the scope of your activities.* It is a mistake to put all your emotional eggs in one corporate basket. A person whose identity relies solely on his position at work becomes too dependent on his success or failure in this one sphere. As Clark Kerr, Chancellor of the University of California at Berkeley, put it: "I would urge each individual to avoid total involvement in any organization: to seek to whatever extent lies within his power to limit each group to the minimum control necessary for performance of essential functions; to struggle against the effort to absorb; to lend his energies to many organizations and give himself completely to none."

11

THE HERD INSTINCT

Man is by nature and training a social animal. To survive in prehistoric times he had to capture wild game. This entailed the formation of disciplined hunting teams. To defend himself against the onslaught of neighboring tribes he formed tightly knit armies. To create a culture, to hold ritual ceremonies and build megalithic monuments he had to accept close cooperation with all his kinsmen. A similar, if not greater, degree of social integration is required today to build roads, run community welfare groups, govern nations and create vast industrial empires. We live in a world that requires enormous cooperation to keep things going and precious little obstruction to bring them to a grinding halt. From this cooperative endeavor we derive our greatest triumphs and our most bitter disappointments, our moments of ecstasy and our moments of frustration and resentment. Most executives when asked reported that a

large proportion of their stress at work came from interpersonal conflicts, from personality clashes, misunderstand-
ings and breakdowns in communication.

In childhood we are aggravated as much by a construction toy that will not fit together as we are by a parent who
refuses to do what we want. When we reach adulthood the
position changes and we are far more likely to be frustrated by people than by things. We will accept with resignation the photocopier that breaks down but become
exceedingly annoyed with a secretary who returns ten
minutes late from lunch. Success in business lies in the
ability to cooperate with others and derive the best from
them. One firm of industrial psychologists estimates that
job success is only fifteen percent due to technical skill and
ability and eighty-five percent due to personality qualities
which make for harmonious working relationships with
other people. Yet in practice most businessmen show less
understanding of the psychology of handling people than
the local bartender.

We all need to belong, and the great pandemic psychological disease of the age is a feeling of alienation. This
probably stems from increasing social mobility, repeated
job and home transfers, smaller family units which are
increasingly inward looking, the steady decline in group
activities such as church-going, community singing and
dancing, and the constant use of the automobile, which
effectively isolates people from their fellows. We may try
to satisfy our frustrated affiliation needs by participating in
encounter groups, rock festivals, drug parties and pro-
miscuous sex, but unless these group activities introduce us
to people with whom we share a genuine mutual interest,
we are likely to finish up feeling more lonely than ever
before. So to satisfy these thwarted longings we turn increasingly to the nuclear family unit, on which we often

place excessive and unreasonable demands, and to our work, which is, for many people, the only sphere in which they can identify themselves as belonging to a close supportive group in which they feel both liked and needed.

The need to experience this strong sense of belonging is more marked in some people than others. It is a quality that shapes our character, albeit in a way that is often masked by the interplay of other personality characteristics. The behavior of dependent people with high affiliation needs, for example, is characterized by a constant desire to please, cooperate, agree and assist. Dependent people with low affiliation, on the other hand, tend to evade, concede, relinquish and withdraw. In the same way a dominant executive with high affiliation needs is prone to advise, lead, coordinate and coax, while those with low affiliation needs tend to analyze, criticize and judge.

We all share the basic need to belong, and the success of any cooperative venture depends on harnessing this drive and fostering harmonious group activity without sacrificing the irreplaceable enthusiasm and creative flair of the individuals involved. The British Socony-Vacuum Oil Company once issued a booklet to employees which read:

> *No room for virtuosos*—Except in certain research assignments, few specialists in a large company ever work alone. There is little room for virtuoso performances. Business is so complex, even in its non-technical aspects, that no one man can master all of it; to do his job, therefore, he must be able to work with other people.

This plea for group unity is sound enough, but it overlooks the fact that ideas, enthusiasm and drive issue from individuals rather than organizations. Corporations are dead, static structures. Like carefully designed, well-oiled machinery, they are only as effective as the men operating them. Of themselves they cannot create a single novel idea, sell a product, or breathe fire into a dormant venture.

Political leaders have always counseled their supporters: "United we stand, divided we fall." Primitive tribesmen are equally aware of the value of group solidarity and have a profound belief that while as individuals they may be weak and ineffectual, as a united tribe they are invested with superhuman power. The same concept of synergistic action applies in industry. It is typified by the confidential memo sent to executives by Maxey Jarman, head of Genesco, the giant textile, clothing and department stores conglomerate: "Two plus two = five or more." But this applies only when the participants share the same aims. If they do not see eye to eye, the chances are that the product of the joint action will be represented by the sum two minus two = zero.

When man cooperates he always does so for a reason. He may band with others to build a house, make music or fight to defend his country. Once this corporate goal is reached the group disbands. Now we have made such a fetish of cooperation that we frequently join groups just for the pleasure and security of belonging even if its aims are alien or so ill-defined that they cannot be clearly discerned. If the effectiveness of corporate activity is to be increased, and the incidence of intra-group conflict reduced, it is essential to see that as far as possible the group shares the same aims and aspirations. We must endeavor to create institutions where the welfare of the individual is in accordance with the welfare of the group. Then when one benefits all will benefit. Managers must be encouraged not to cling to power but to radiate it. Then they will enhance the status of others and increase the potency of the group rather than merely advance their own self-interest. Wher-

ever possible corporate goals should be chosen in preference to purely individual goals and cooperation fostered
rather than intra-group competition.

There are an infinite number of ways of stimulating
group loyalty. In America it may be done by circulating
eulogistic company magazines and holding lavish company
dinners; in England by sporting the company tie, and in
Japan by wearing the company uniform and singing the
company song. These methods can be effective when carefully used. There are, however, four other techniques for
achieving group unity which are somewhat more subtle
and far more fundamental. They are:

1. The establishment of clear-cut communal aims.
2. The delineation of well-defined group boundaries and the
   establishment of a strict intra-group hierarchy.
3. The provision of strong leadership.
4. The definition, or if necessary creation, of a potentially
   threatening outside group.

Leadership is essential to the continued existence of a
group. Without it an organization becomes like a ship
without a rudder. Unfortunately, in the name of democ-
racy we sometimes struggle to achieve corporate leadership,
participative management or government by consensus.
This is all too often a pretty, flower-lined garden path
which leads to group incompetence and endless frustration
and stress for individuals who are powerless to act unless
they first obtain majority consent.

When an infantry officer is pinned down by enemy fire
at the edge of a wood, he sizes up the situation and decides
he can take several courses of action. He can lie low until
nightfall, when he can beat a retreat under cover of darkness. He can send a runner to reestablish contact with

battalion headquarters and request reinforcements or covering artillery fire. Alternatively he can mount an attack on his own. But if he attacks, which of three obvious routes should he take? Should he get the machine gun forces to provide covering fire, or should he be content to advance behind a smokescreen? If he holds an on-the-spot referendum and waits to get the unanimous agreement of all the members of his platoon the battle will inevitably be lost. A leader must be free to make decisions without having constantly to refer either to the group or to his hierarchical superiors.

The natural leader inspires confidence and gains support with little effort on his part. When discipline has to be exerted, he knows instinctively how best it should be applied. He recognizes the individuals who are more amenable to group influence and leaves them to be admonished by their peers. Those who respond to authority he deals with privately. Those with psychopathic tendencies he isolates so that they cause the minimum possible disruption to the smooth running of the group. Moreover he feels sufficiently secure that he does not need to run away from personal criticism. Many executives suffer tension because they do not feel free to criticize their boss. Others will do so in a snide way, or in a way more damaging to the group, by complaining about him to subordinates. Yet, providing the prime object of the criticism is to advance the welfare of the organization rather than to score over the individual, such criticism helps to clear the air and is rarely taken amiss. William B. Given, Jr., Chairman of the American Brake Shoe Corporation, when asked how bosses should be criticized, said: "In about the same manner as you yourself would want to be criticized by a subordinate. Nobody particularly enjoys criticism. Yet if you feel something the boss is doing or failing to do cramps your performance or that of someone else in your department, this means that he is cramping his performance, too. You should be able to find an acceptable way to discuss it with him. Actually this is not so difficult as it may seem; he may take it as a compliment that you feel free to criticize."

The philosopher Herbert Spencer recognized that the formation of groups entailed not only the establishment of an "in" group, but also the recognition of rival "out" groups. In his *Principles of Ethics* he described the process by which we develop amity for our own group, and enmity for rival groups. This emotional polarization has a powerful survival value for groups struggling to exist in either the primeval rain forests or the modern business jungle. As Darwin pointed out, "When two tribes of primeval man, living in the same country, come into competition, the tribe including the greater number of courageous, sympathetic and faithful members would succeed better and conquer the others."

To a certain extent we can improve our social skills by attending encounter groups. When properly run these sessions help to increase self-awareness and make us more sensitive to the behavior of others and quicker to understand the processes which facilitate or inhibit group interaction. On an individual level we can foster group interaction by adopting the following tactics:

- *Always look at things from the other person's point of view.* As Henry Ford said, "If there is any one secret of success, it lies in the ability to get the other person's point of view and see things from his angle as well as your own." This golden rule is reiterated in a remarkably similar way in the scriptures of all the world's major religions. The *Undanavarga* instructs Buddhists: "Hurt not others in ways that you yourself would find hurtful." "This is the sum of duty," the *Mahabharat* tells Brahmins: "Do naught unto others which would cause pain if done to you." Followers of Islam are told, "No one of you is a believer until he desires for his brother that which he desires for himself." The New Testament tells Christians, "All things whatsoever ye would that men should do to you, do ye even so to them." And the Talmud tells Jews, "What is hateful to you, do not to your fellow man. That is the entire Law: all the rest is commentary."

- *Show tact and courtesy.* The principles of good manners have been developed and refined over the years as a result of extensive clinical trials. Experience has shown that they are the finest ways of oiling the wheels of social intercourse. As Edmund Burke observed, "Manners are what vex or soothe, corrupt or purify, exalt or debase." The successful executive is often pictured as a tough, ruthless and uncaring character. But this stereotype is far from the truth, for even in the world of commerce, tact invariably succeeds where bluster and bullying fail. There is an old fable which tells how the sun and the wind set out to contest their strength. The wind, to prove his supremacy, pointed to an elderly man and said: "To show my strength I'll whip that old man's coat from his back." So he raised a gale and then a hurricane, but the harder he blew the more firmly the man drew his coat around him. Finally the wind gave up the struggle and the sun came out and shone brightly down. In a few moments the man took off his coat and started to mop his brow. "See," said the sun, "more can be achieved by gentleness and warmth than by all the fury and force." As Claudianus, the last of the great Latin poets, said, "Power can do by gentleness that which violence fails to accomplish: and calmness best enforces the imperial mandate."

- *Develop mutual trust.* Nothing is more damaging to interpersonal relationships than lack of trust. As Confucius said, "If you suspect a man do not employ him: if you employ him, do not suspect him."

- *Praise frequently, condemn rarely.* If you try to find the good in people rather than the bad, you will invariably find what you are looking for. Most people appreciate the occasional compliment, which provides useful outside confirmation of their importance and worth. But the praise needs to be carefully judged. If it is too effusive the receiver may think it is phony or will feel guilty because it is not warranted and will worry how it can best be returned. As Roger Severson, a professor of educational psychology has said, "When you compliment someone, you must not exceed that person's tolerance level. If you go to extremes, the person you're praising will say: 'That's not really me—that makes me feel like a fraud.' "

  Reproofs must be given with equal care; preferably in private and in a way which does not damage the individual's self-esteem. One of the best techniques is to make a sympathetic presentation of the facts, then ask the individual for his personal views on the situation, what caused it, and how it can be prevented from happening again. Having heard his version of the story, suggest a trial period during which his remedies can be put to the test, followed by a second meeting at which the situation can be reviewed.

- *Express good humor and tranquility.* The most valuable assets in any business negotiations are a cool head and a warm heart. Violent arguments are always risky. It is a poor bargain to win an argument but lose a valued customer or friend. Executives must strive to acquire the qualities of calmness, patience and cheerfulness, for if they are to work in peace with others, they must first learn to live in peace with themselves. As Balzac said, "To be boldly tranquil, to speak little, and to digest without effort are absolutely necessary to grandeur of mind and of presence, or to the proper development of genius."

12

A VIVID IMAGINATION

Imagination is the mental faculty which most sharply distinguishes us from other animals. It is the process that permits us to form ideas and images which are not directly related to the happenings of the moment; the gift which enables us to achieve prestigious feats of creative and conceptual thought. Without its aid businessmen would be powerless to create new products, anticipate future market trends or estimate the effectiveness of projected advertising campaigns.

Imaginative flights of fancy and daydreams can also be used as a means of temporary escape from the pressures and problems of day-to-day living, and as an explorative way of preparing for the future and testing out possible courses of action. This is a natural and wholly commendable pattern of behavior providing the gap between fantasy and reality does not grow too great. If it does, we run the risk of suffering disillusionment when our real selves fail to live up to our idealized self-image. Disappointment must arise if our achievements fall far short of our soaring dreams and we must experience despair if the real world is colorless, flat and stale, and not vivid and varied as we picture in our mind's eye. We laugh at Frederick Rolfe for imagining himself as Pope in *Hadrian the Seventh*, for his reveries are so far removed from reality; but we admire the prescience of Winston Churchill who at the age of twenty-six pictured himself as leader in his only novel, *Savrola*. We can indulge in what Arnold Bennett describes as the "agreeable deceptions" of ambition and hope; but while we can afford to let them kid us a little, we must not allow them to cheat us a lot.

Imagination is a powerful two-edged tool which needs to be handled with care in case it damages the hand which wields it. A faculty which can conjure up constructive ideas and positive concepts can equally well invoke specters of doom and despair. With a vivid imagination we can all too easily dwell on yesterday's defeats and tomorrow's anticipated terrors, as well as the problems of the day. This is a source of stress peculiar to man. Animals will react instantly to danger in their immediate environment, but will relax the moment the peril is past. Man, on the other hand, will often show an anxiety reaction weeks before an anticipated crisis arrives and then, instead of relaxing when the crisis is over, will continue to relive the event in all its harrowing detail. A herd of zebra will flee when chased by a hungry lion, but once one of its weaker members is captured and the lion's appetite temporarily assuaged, the remainder of the herd will contentedly settle down to graze, often within a few feet of the feeding lion. In a similar situation we would remain for hours in a state of quivering terror, empathizing with our friend, visualizing his suffering, and anticipating our personal agony should we be next on the list. This tendency is a potent source of stress. Experiments in psychology laboratories have shown that the *anticipation* of a stressful event can give rise to more anxiety (as measured by the output of hydrocortisone) than the actual *experience* of the event. If we are to escape psychosomatic illness we need to keep our imagination tightly under control.

When a man with a normal grip strength of 101 pounds was hypnotized and given the suggestion that he was exceedingly strong, he somehow found the strength to exert a grip of 142 pounds. When the experiment was repeated and he was told he was weak, his hand strength fell to a puny 29 pounds. This gives some idea of the power of the imagination over our performance. "As a man thinketh in his heart, so is he." Émile Coué, pioneer founder of a clinic for healing by hypnosis, used to give his patients a telling illustration of the power of the imagination. Nobody finds any difficulty walking along a foot-wide plank when it is placed on the ground, he would say, and yet nearly everyone would be unable to traverse the plank if it were suspended sixty feet up between two tall buildings. What is the difference? Merely that in the first place you imagine it is easy to traverse the plank, in the second you picture yourself falling. Behavior follows the furrows plowed by the imagination. If at a critical stage in a tennis match we imagine we are going to lose a vital service point, we invariably serve a double fault. As Coué demonstrated repeatedly in his clinic in Nancy, "Our actions spring not from our Will but from our Imaginations." Achieve control over your thoughts and you immediately achieve a large degree of mastery over your actions. Anyone who can exercise control over his imagination can reduce his level of anxiety. Chronic worriers are made, not born. Worry is a habit acquired by learning and reinforced by constant practice. In any day we have the choice of dwelling on the pleasant aspects of life, or brooding on the sad. As Frederick Langbridge said, "Two men look out through the same bars: One sees the mud, and one the stars." The choice is ours, the upward look or the dejected, downcast glance. The decision is far reaching in its effects for it orders not only our conduct today but also our experience tomorrow. We are creatures of habit and by constant repetition we acquire emotional attitudes. Through practice we become habitually cheerful or glum, optimistic or depressed, relaxed or tense, confident or nervous. If we choose, we can fill our minds with the negative emotions of grief, remorse, anger, resentment, and fear, or concentrate on the positive affects of cheerfulness and hope. We will be visited by occasional disappointments, failures and setbacks but there's no need to make them prolonged house guests. As an old Chinese proverb puts it, "You cannot prevent the birds of sorrow from flying over your head, but you can prevent them from building nests in your hair." Unpleasant memories will fade away providing they are not constantly recalled to mind. We do not have to make any conscious effort to forget: time alone will sponge the slate clean providing we halt the process of constant recollection. Remembering is an active process, forgetting is passive. We would avoid a prolific source of stress if we allowed the past to bury its mistakes. As the Victorian doggerel puts it: "Many a trouble would break like a bubble . . . Did we not rehearse it and tenderly nurse it." Many real and all imaginary problems would disappear if we did not constantly refabricate them in our mind.

Psychiatrists have coined the term "free-floating anxiety" to describe a persistent mood of worry, unrelated to any outside cause. This habitual emotional tension can be so strong that it dominates a person's every action and thought. Just as the cheerful extrovert looks at life through rose-colored glasses, so the sufferer from free-floating anxiety peers at the world through a miasma of gloom. He sets out to find trouble and is rarely disappointed. He is hypochondriacal about his health and invariably produces enough psychosomatic sickness to justify his deepest fears. In business, instead of communicating to his subordinates messages of confidence and success, he transmits an air of pessimism and defeat. Verbally he is generally not the best of communicators. Experiments have shown that individuals under stress are more likely to show signs of flustered speech, repetitions and omissions, stuttering and incomplete sentences, defects which make their communication seventeen percent less effective than those with low anxiety ratings. The perpetually anxious individual is also more likely to panic under stress and to exhibit specific fears and phobias.

Even the most successful executives are not immune to petty fears. Queen Elizabeth I was not afraid of death but was terrified of visits to her dentist; Cromwell had to be taken to the doctor by his wife, and Disraeli was so afraid of cold water that he would stand under the shower and wait for his wife to turn on the cold tap. Fears such as these are commonplace. A study of a group of three thousand Americans showed that forty-one percent feared speaking in public, thirty-two percent feared heights, twenty-two percent insects and bugs and twenty-two percent deep water. Others admitted to a dread of open spaces (agoraphobia); closed spaces (claustrophobia); blood (haematophobia); cats (ailourophobia); flying (acrophobia) or the dark (nyctophobia). These phobias may be trivial or completely incapacitating. When an otherwise successful manager is terrified of entering a plane or speaking in public, his life is severely curtailed and he is bound to experience stress whenever he is forced to tackle these tasks. Fortunately these fears can generally be mastered. The simplest way of doing this is by a process of direct confrontation. There is an old Irish legend which asserts that if you run away from a ghost it will continue chasing after you, but if you run toward it, it disappears. The same is true of phobias. If you avoid confronting them you heighten their imagined powers. If you successfully face up to them they lose their power to terrify. As Ralph Waldo Emerson said, "Do the thing you fear and the death of fear is certain."

Most of the great British orators have had to conquer overwhelming stage fright at the outset of their careers. Lloyd George confessed that when he first stood up to speak in public, "My tongue clove to the roof of my mouth; and, at first, I could hardly get out a word." Disraeli fared little better, and said that he would rather have delivered a cavalry charge than deliver his maiden speech in the House of Commons; while Charles Parnell, the Irish rebel leader, admitted that he was so nervous when he first addressed a crowd that he clenched his fists so tightly his nails drew blood. If these men had not had the courage to face up to their early fears they would never have achieved their eminence or their reputation for eloquent, persuasive oratory.

A similar forthright approach can be used to overcome the fear of flying, which is said to affect at least nine million Americans in the managerial income brackets. Some are terrified at the thought of leaving the ground. Others have learned to overcome their unreasoned terror with the help of "Flying without Fear," an organization which helps people to face up to their fears by a process of gradual acclimatization. Early meetings are held in airline terminal buildings so that group members can gain a relatively stress-free introduction to aircraft, airports and airline personnel. When they are confident in these situations they hold meetings in stationary aircraft, and only when this can be achieved without anxiety are they taken on a forty-five minute jet flight where their fears are allayed by group discussions and the practice of special relaxation exercises. In this way the acrophobic ghosts are slowly put to rout.

The same behavioral techniques can be used to conquer other phobias. The method is basically one of systematic deconditioning. Like Pavlov's dogs our present responses depend to a very large extent on our past experience. If we are conditioned to expect to be afraid when we enter a plane or stand up to give an after-dinner speech, we are bound to react with an anxiety response when these stressful events occur. This reinforces the response. If we can manage to stay relaxed when we are faced with the threatening situation, we weaken the strength of the previously conditioned response and in time attenuate and even extinguish the fear reaction. This can be achieved by preparing a hierarchy of fears from the least threatening to the most terrifying, and then tackling the phobia stage by stage. Thus, in the case of a fear of cats the first step in the hierarchy may be to imagine a cat walking into the room, the next to look at a picture of a kitten or handle a piece of fur and the final step to cradle a live cat in your arms. Progress along the hierarchy is made only when it is possible to tackle the preceding stage without evoking a fear response.

Other techniques can be developed to conquer nonspecific worries. Four valuable strategies are:

- *Strive to live in the present.* Abraham Maslow noted that successful, well-adjusted people have the ability to be "lost in the present." They are so absorbed in what they are doing that they forget the cares of the past, and have no time to think about the hypothetical difficulties of the future. The time most people spend in worrying about the past would be sufficient, if properly applied, to eradicate the problems of the present. Besides, we only create unnecessary anxiety if we try to carry tomorrow's burdens today. We can reduce our load of worry if we make a strict practice of living a day at a time. This is a pressure which even the most timorous can tolerate. As Robert Louis Stevenson said, "Anyone can carry his burden, however hard, until nightfall." Living in the present will improve our concentration and also increase our creativity and happiness. If we are forever looking to the concepts of yesterday we are hardly likely to produce innovations appropriate to the needs of today; and if we are constantly postponing our enjoyment of life until a hoped-for tomorrow we will fail to savor the pleasures of the moment.

- *Learn to be more spontaneous.* Personality studies show that the well-integrated person is spontaneous in his actions. He is not hedged in by the routines of the past or by anxieties about the future. Such people are sufficiently sure of their knowledge and ability to do things their way, to think on their feet, to run their businesses by the seat of their pants rather than by the managerial rule book.

- *Dispel doubt by purposeful action.* The timid exhaust themselves in the endless debate "Shall I, shan't I? . . . Dare I, daren't I?" They vacillate rather than risk making a mistake. But life is never without risks and the person who is afraid to make a mistake usually ends up by making nothing. You can never learn to swim unless you are bold enough to enter the water. And the only way to banish fears, doubts and crippling indecision is to make a firm step forward. As Shakespeare warned, "Our doubts are traitors, and make us lose the good we oft might win by fearing to attempt."

• *Cultivate equanimity.* Dr. Irvine Page, a well-known heart specialist, suggests that the best way to avoid heart attacks is through the "achievement of equanimity." Some men achieve this intellectually through developing a positive philosophy of life. "Others," he says, "achieve equanimity emotionally, through a belief in beauty, in ideals, in unselfishness. They let the annoyances of life pass in one side and out the other." Ruskin suggested that we can cultivate serenity by building up a treasure house of restful thoughts: "Bright fancies, satisfied memories, noble histories, faithful sayings . . . which care cannot disturb, nor pain make gloomy, nor poverty take away from us." Whatever technique we use to attain it, equanimity becomes a valuable antidote to stress. It is the emotional state most directly opposed to free-floating anxiety. When it is firmly established as our fundamental and habitual mood we can relax in the sure knowledge that whatever comes along to disturb our peace of mind will be purely temporary.

13

MARITAL STRESS

In 1964 the British Institute of Directors carried out a study of the incidence of stress among their members. They found that problems at home caused nearly as much stress as tensions at work. Most of the executives they questioned were forced to admit that their marriages were not as happy as they would have liked. A later review of three thousand men attending the Institute's Medical Center showed that sixteen percent of managers had marriages which were patently unhappy. This gives rise to considerable emotional strain.

Accountants exhibit a marked increase in their blood-cholesterol levels and blood-clotting times when they are working under pressure toward the end of the fiscal year. But these potentially harmful stress reactions are doubled when they go through a period of domestic upheaval such as a divorce. Marital conflict can be a cause of more than the purely metaphorical heartache. Dr. R. H. Rahe confirmed this when he carried out his inquiry into the stress caused by crises in people's lives. He found that fights with the boss, changes of job, retirement and getting fired were frequent causes of stress and a common contributing factor to heart attacks and other stress disorders. To these events he gave a stress rating of 23, 36, 45 and 47 respectively. Far more damaging were the crises which occurred in the home, such as separation and divorce—which, analysis showed, merited ratings of 65 and 73.

As well as affecting our health, domestic stress also impairs our working efficiency. This is clearly seen with airline pilots. Dr. Lionel Haward, Reader in Clinical Psychology at England's Surrey University, reckons that over seventy percent of airline pilots suffer stress from marital problems which are severe enough to affect their flying efficiency. With the aid of tests on flight simulators he has demonstrated that when they are involved in domestic crises pilots are less vigilant, less responsive to stimuli and more prone to make mistakes such as failing to keep the plane on course, maintain the right height and angle of approach during landing or to switch fuel tanks at the appropriate time. This is confirmed by airline authorities in Holland who carry out psychological autopsies after crashes to try to assess the psychological state of the pilot at the time. They find that many incidents of pilot error can be traced to emotional stress.

The airline pilot is particularly prone to get enmeshed in domestic conflict because he is frequently away from home, and spends days, and all too often nights, in the company of young, attractive stewardesses. The businessman suffers because he devotes so much of his life to his work. President of Texas Instruments J. Fred Bucy told reporters that he starts his working day at 7:30 A.M., takes home a minimum of three briefcases of papers and works on them until "past midnight" every day. Work schedules of this nature may be intensely satisfying, but leave little time for family life. Many executives are quite aware that they allow their work to take precedence over their home. Sociologists Peter Willmott and Michael Young studied the lives of two thousand people living in and around London and found that two-thirds of the executives they questioned recognized that their business commitments interfered with their marriages and home life. Others deny that they give a disproportionate amount of time and attention to their work, but might be forced to change their mind if they tried to find honest answers to the following questions:

1. When asked by a stranger at a party to identify yourself, are you more likely to reply:
   a. "I'm in the advertising department at Marshall Field's."
   b. "I live in Evanston with my wife and three children."
2. Under normal circumstances is the time you spend at work thinking about your family more or less than the time you spend at home thinking about your work?
3. If both you and your wife are reasonably content with your current standard of living and you are offered a change of job would you choose:
   a. A sideways promotion which involved no change in salary or status but enabled you to spend more time with your family.
   b. A promotion which gave you an extra $5000 a year but meant that you would have to work longer hours and spend a number of days away from home.

Many women find it hard to understand that through work a man derives an important source of security, comradeship, status and self-esteem. These are needs which tradition says a woman should satisfy through her home, family and marital bond. She marries a man to satisfy these needs and to enjoy his company and affection, then finds that he spends a large part of his time in the embrace of a rival concern. She feels cheated when her husband commits "corporate bigamy" and does not feel adequately compensated when he assures her that he is doing it all for her sake and that of the children. She knows this is not true. This schism is particularly noticeable in the lives of ambitious young men who by dint of hard work have achieved a succession of rapid promotions. The British Institute of Management examined the marriages of a number of these men and found that the wife of a young executive finds it increasingly difficult to understand the satisfactions he achieves from his work. This failure to understand his satisfactions, his driving ambitions, frustrations and recurrent problems causes a rift which, according to the Institute's report, imposes "considerable strain on the stability of a large number of marriages." This strain would be lessened if wives would only show a greater interest in their husbands' work and if husbands took equal pains to satisfy this curiosity.

The increasing emancipation of women has swelled the number of working wives who are now, like their husbands, no longer dependent on marriage for the satisfaction of their natural yearning for status, security and self-esteem. This change in the housewife's traditional role has undoubtedly eased her lot, but has increased the stresses placed upon her mate. A survey of marriages in Ontario, Canada, where both husband and wife are working showed that while the wives expressed greater satisfaction with their marriages and lives, their husbands reported less satisfaction with their work, lives and marriages, experienced greater job pressures, and suffered more physical and psychological stress.

Other problems arise because many people today have greatly increased expectations of marriage. The wife who at one time might have been satisfied with a marriage which provided her with a roof over her head, adequate food and clothing, and a tolerably considerate spouse, now asks her husband for intellectual stimulation, close companionship, shared values, deep romantic love, and repeated ecstatic and varied sexual pleasures. If she fails to get them she may decide to look elsewhere. This was a major finding of a survey conducted by *The New York Times*, which showed that a major factor in the increased rate of divorce in the United States was the "revolution of rising expectations." It is natural that a male executive who devotes a large amount of his time to his work should find it difficult, if not impossible, to meet these greatly amplified demands. The stress this causes depends to a large extent on the tolerance and understanding of his wife. As William H. Whyte observes in his study *The Wives of Management*, an executive's wife is "good by *not* doing things—by *not* complaining when her husband works late; by *not* fussing when a transfer is coming up; by *not* engaging in any controversial activity." Some wives feel overstretched by their role as a senior executive's wife, others grossly under-employed. Some are content to accept their supportive role, while others are constantly struggling to assert their dominance or narrow the gap between their desire for a close, exclusive conjugal relationship and the reality of the separateness of their lives.

The executive whose wife is discontented with her lot is bound to suffer stress. Studies have shown that when a wife suffers prolonged feelings of depression or guilt her husband has an above-average chance of having a coronary attack. As Dr. Beverly Daily, who first made this observation, said, "To many men the greatest stress in their lives must be at home where they are continually striving to 'make things better' in the misguided hope that it will improve their wives' attitude toward life." But this rarely works. A mink coat and an elegant second car do not satisfy the justified demands of a frustrated wife. The only real solution is for an executive to choose a wife whose personality is compatible with the demands of his career. As he invariably makes his choice before his career takes shape, and for totally different reasons, it seems inevitable that in later life many executives should find themselves sadly mismatched. A short while ago the London Business School carried out a small study of executive marriages in which they classified the personalities of each partner according to the presence or absence of four characteristic drives: Achievement (A), Dominance (B), Autonomy (C), and Submission (D). It was found that most executive marriages fall into the BD category, in which an ambitious husband is married to a caring wife. This is generally a sound basis for a managerial mating since the roles of both partners are clearly defined and compatible, the husband acting as breadwinner, the wife as homemaker, hostess, comforter and undemanding friend. The next most common patterns are AA and CD marriages. In the AA pairings both partners want the satisfaction of their own careers, but since they are not loners they share within their union a considerable degree of intimacy and warmth. These marriages provide a less stable background for the husband's career since his wife has less time to devote to his emotional needs and material comforts. The home is often chaotic, and housework, darning and cooking are generally relegated to low places in her list of priorities. In CD marriages the men are independent and find it annoying to be the object of their wives' constant attention while the wives, finding that their care and devotion is spurned, feel both unwanted and unappreciated. Stress is lessened in these cases if each partner can become aware of the roles he or she plays, and the conflict which arises from their interaction.

There are many other ways to reduce the stress of marital discord. Several of these techniques can be singled out as being particularly applicable to executives and their wives:

- *Learn to cope with anger.* A degree of hostility is present from time to time in all healthy relationships. Marriages do not break down because people have rows, but because they do not know how to handle the fights which occur. Damage frequently occurs because aggressive feelings are not expressed but bottled up. As Dr. George Bach says in *The Intimate Enemy: How to Fight Fair in Love and Marriage*: "The danger of a nuclear explosion hovers over every non-fighting marriage." The trick is to learn how to give vent to anger in a non-hurtful way. Dr. Bach suggests that this can be done by limiting arguments to current events, by avoiding throwing up old arguments, by refusing to use absolute terms like "You always do this" or "You never do that," and by taking care to attack the action rather than the person. During every row the question should be asked: "What am I trying to achieve?" If the answer is to inflict pain or exact punishment the fight should be stopped. The intention should be to tell the other partner why you are hurt or angry, and then try and work out a mutually acceptable solution to the problem.

- *Accentuate the positive.* It is a mistake to focus too much attention on the problem areas of a marriage.

Far better to concentrate on its positive qualities and hope that as these grow the relationship's other, less desirable characteristics will wane.

- *Plan a regular schedule of shared activities.* Since most executives lead hectic lives it is wise for them to set aside some regular times to devote to their wives—a ritual pre-dinner drink, a weekend in the country, a regular game of golf or bridge, dinner parties, theater trips and birthday treats. Time should also be found for showing affection and making love, a pastime sadly neglected by many businessmen who are generally far better bread-winners than bedwinners. One survey of ten thousand marriages showed that while ninety-nine percent of wives were satisfied with their husbands' earning capacity, only two percent thought they were getting the best out of sex. As a result a quarter of the wives were going outside their marriages for sexual satisfaction. As Robert Chester, the sociologist who conducted the survey, said, "Many wives would rather see their husbands less masculine in the traditional sense and more human." In the boardroom a man may feel he needs to be tough and abrasive, but in the bedroom he needs to be tender, gentle and caring.

- *Respect your partner's privacy.* While it is important for married couples to share a wide range of activities, it is equally necessary for them to enjoy periods of complete and absolute privacy. The marriage bond should not be tied so tightly that we feel trapped and claustrophobic. Partners in even the happiest of marriages need to feel free;

those in less successful unions need an even greater margin of freedom and autonomy. In our march to achieve togetherness, we must not deny our need to exist as individuals, nor must we interpret as rejection our partner's understandable need for occasional periods of solitude.

- *Decide how to allocate the family budget.* A surprising amount of marital conflict arises from financial arguments. These are rarely related to an overall shortage of funds, but more often to the way the available cash is spent. A wife, to assure herself that she is respected and loved, may need to acquire diamonds and furs. Her husband, to boost his sense of security, may need to swell his investment portfolio. These incompatible goals can be reconciled only by establishing a mutually acceptable budget and by realizing that these financial squabbles are matters less of money than differing attitudes, emotions and goals.

14

THE SECURE LIFE

Life in the higher echelons of the business world can never be secure. Each week is full of unforeseen perils and agonizing uncertainties. But then it is these hazards that give a businessman's life its piquancy and appeal. A man who places a high premium on security tends to opt for a nine-to-five job with little or no responsibility. Either consciously or unconsciously he heeds the warning, "If you can't stand the heat, stay out of the kitchen." The executive, on the other hand, like a circus artist, actually revels in the excitement of taking calculated risks, and while others tremble on the ground below he walks the high wire with a steady, confident step. This willingness and ability to take risks is one of his chief characteristics and major assets. It is this ability which makes him a successful executive, a fact we acknowledge when we describe his commercial undertakings as business *ventures*.

Freud did not tell the whole story when he tried to explain all human behavior on the basis of the pleasure principle. We do undoubtedly derive pleasure from the relief of tension, but equally well we derive challenge and excitement from the stimulation of tension. After coitus, when our sexual needs are satisfied, we sink back into a state of contented relaxation. This condition Freud likened to the state of a suckling infant "sinking back satisfied from the breast and falling asleep with flushed cheeks and a blissful smile." Delightful though these moments of contentment are, we would find a life of unrelieved satisfaction and satiation unbearably dull and uninspired. We need the stimulus of adventure to spur us on. Sir Ernest Shackleton got hundreds of replies to the small advertisement he placed in *The* [London] *Times* in 1900:

Men wanted for Hazardous Journey. Small wages, bitter cold, long months of complete darkness, constant danger, safe return doubtful. Honor and recognition in case of success.

Many men saw in this challenge a heaven-sent opportunity to escape from the dull routine of their lives.

Fortunately we achieve a total escape from danger only when we are in the womb or tomb, and in the first case life has hardly begun, while in the second it has gone forever. The art is to introduce into our lives sufficient uncertainty to provide the optimum spur to endeavor without overstepping the mark and suffering an excess of stressful insecurity.

As one industrialist said: "The day I'm secure, I'm dead." At one time the hazards and uncertainties of everyday life inevitably kept us on the *qui vive*. Now many people are beginning to suffer the lethargy and ennui of having too little adventure in their lives. Recognizing this, many try to replace the deficiency and restore the balance by indulging in what the travel agencies refer to as "risk recreation." Surveys show that some of the fastest-growing pastimes are those which provide a measure of danger and thrill—sky diving, mountaineering, canoeing and hang gliding. It is also interesting to note the uncanny tendency of executives, once they have achieved financial security, to go out of their way to place it all in jeopardy. Many exchange the excitement of commercial risk-taking for the synthetic thrill of gambling. Gordon Selfridge, the American who made a fortune by establishing the first department store in London, risked everything and eventually went bankrupt because of his passion for gambling and expensive women. André Citroën, founder of the multimillion French car empire, satisfied his lust for excitement by playing baccarat and once lost $550,000 at a single session. More recently millionaire British store boss Sir Hugh Fraser had to sell nearly £1,500,000 of his shares to meet heavy betting losses at race tracks and casinos. These men craved excitement. Once their businesses were established and failed to provide them with sufficient challenge and adventure, they were forced to get their thrills elsewhere.

Men with ambition, but a relatively low tolerance for risk-taking, are naturally attracted to the security of a large organization. Here they have the comforting assurances of generous pension schemes, company loans, health benefits and the promise, if they are ever needed, of generous unemployment compensation. They are pampered by the parent company, and in times of stress can always turn to a higher authority for support. Paternalism of this kind can go too far. A child, or junior executive, who is never allowed to take full responsibility for his actions will never achieve maturity and will always be haunted by the nagging anxiety that if adversity strikes and he is deprived of his protecting father figures, he will be unable to stand on his own two feet. During the Battle of Crécy Edward III wisely allowed his son to enter the thick of the fray. When a knight asked for troops to protect the young prince the king refused, saying, "Let the boy win his spurs." In the home and in business we need to provide more opportunity for young men to gain their spurs. Several executives I questioned admitted to feeling insecure. They suffered stress because they feared they might lose their jobs as a result of layoffs, takeovers, mergers or company dissolutions. They worried whether they would be able in the future to earn enough to meet their financial commitments, or were concerned lest ill health should deprive them to their ability to earn a living.

Persistent worries like these show a basic lack of self-confidence. We look for security in a job or in material possessions, but the only security worth having comes from within. We escape anxiety only if we have the calm assurance that we will be equal to whatever demands may be placed upon us. This quiet, inner strength can be acquired. It can be fostered by practicing the following techniques:

- *Learn to live with little.* As critic Joseph Wood Crutch observes, "Security depends not so much upon how much you have as upon how much you can do without." If we feel we must have the comforts of a luxury home, the services of a secretary to organize our day, a limousine to take us from place to place, and a bottle of Scotch for relaxation in the evening, we must also experience anxiety at the realization that at any time we may lose one or all of these props. The fewer our wants the less our

risk of deprivation. Epictetus, the Greek philosopher, lived by this philosophy. He was contented,
free and untrammeled by care and worries; yet he
had no money, possessions or home. "Only the earth
and heavens and one poor cloak." Having so little
no one could rob him of what he had. As Mao Tse-
tung said, "Obsession with comforts makes men
decadent and spiritually barren. Deprivation, aus-
terity, struggle, make self-reliance."

- *Have a second string to your bow.* Security can be
derived from having carefully prepared contingency
plans. The organizers of an outdoor company picnic
will inevitably be anxiously scanning the skies
when the great day dawns unless they have made
alternative arrangements to hold the event in the
town hall in case of rain.

   Both the pessimist and the astute realist repeatedly ask themselves the question "What can go
wrong?" The pessimist uses this forethought to add
to his air of melancholia; the realist to circumvent
disaster. We have little to fear if we plan fail-safe
devices to protect against every conceivable catas-
trophe. We know then that we can cope, whatever
happens. When it is impossible to eliminate all uncertainty, a useful trick is to ask the question "What
is the worst that can happen?" It is always reassuring to discover that we can survive in even this
extremity.

   The great violinist Ole Bull was once giving a
concert in Paris when his A string snapped. Immediately he transposed the piece and finished the
composition on three strings. That is one of the
secrets of serenity, the knowledge that if misfortune

strikes we have the ability to carry on life with only three strings.

- *Do not put all your eggs in one basket.* The broader-based our resources, the greater our security. Executives whose experience lies in narrowly specialized fields are taking a greater risk than those who have a wide range of skills and are able to turn their hands to any managerial task.

  A further safeguard is to build up a capital reserve which can be used in case of emergency. Many prudent executives draw comfort from the assurance that if they lose their jobs they can always finance a small business of their own.

- *Learn to take risks.* Practice in risk-taking helps to build confidence and dispel anxiety. During the Second World War psychologist Dr. Paul Torrence made a special study of ace U.S. pilots and found that one of their major characteristics was an ability to take risks. This calculated daring improved their performance and far from making them prone to accidents, actually added to their safety. As Dr. Torrence concluded, "Life itself is a risky business. If we spent half as much time learning how to take risks as we spend avoiding them, we wouldn't have so much to fear in life." Security, like happiness, is elusive. We find it only by risking it.

Part III
THE CONTROL OF STRESS

15
THE CLIMATE OF REPOSE

Like the chameleon, man is highly influenced by his surroundings. Entertain him at a candlelit supper with soft, romantic music playing in the background and he will feel in the mood for love. Bombard him with martial music, shouted slogans, brandished fists and waving banners, and his patriotic fervor will be roused possibly to the point where he will be prepared to lay down his life for his country. Such is the sensitivity of human behavior to environmental conditioning.

Oddly enough this behavioral quirk has received little acknowledgment within industry where people are sometimes expected to produce accurate mental work in conditions more suited to a Caribbean folk festival. We encourage millions of people to work in cities, even though we know that in many ways this environment is inimical to prolonged mental work. When interrogated, fifty-two percent of white-collar workers said they found working in London stressful, thirty-five percent because of the tiring journey to and from work, twenty percent because of the noise, eighteen percent because of the pace of city life and sixteen percent because of overcrowding. These employees would almost certainly be happier, and more effective, if they were able to work in a small provincial town. But it should be possible to improve the working environment of large sections of the community without embarking on a massive scheme of job relocation. As a first step a reduction can be made in the general level of environmental noise. This is a common source of annoyance among executives. As a doctor reported to a medical conference, "Noise lowers all our faculties. It clouds judgment and reduces the precision of our actions. It decreases efficiency and drags personality to a lower level: it makes us irritable, pessimistic and grumpy." This has been proved by numerous experiments.

Scientists at Cambridge University carried out tests to determine the effect of noise on mental performance. They gave two groups of volunteers the task of mentally subtracting a series of numbers, the first group working in a quiet environment, the second against a background of noise. The experiment demonstrated, as anticipated, that noise has an adverse effect on the efficiency of work; but it also showed that this effect persists long after the noise has ceased. When the same tests were repeated, with both groups working in a quiet environment, it was found that the performance of the first group improved while that of the second remained the same, showing that the handicap of originally working in a noisy environment had impaired not only the immediate accuracy and speed of their work, but also their long-term ability to learn and benefit from past experience.

With typists and clerical workers it is often possible to make a quantitative assessment of the damage caused by excess noise. One telegraph company, for example, enjoyed a drop in reported clerical errors after reducing the level of noise within their offices. A similar though less easily quantified impairment arises in executive performance. Work which involves detailed analysis and complex decision-making cannot easily be achieved against a background of distracting sound. Attempts to do so produce frustration, irritation and needless fatigue. This is a commonly cited cause of stress among managerial workers, and a frequently overlooked cause of nervous illness. As the late Lord Horder, physician to England's Queen Elizabeth, said: "Noise wears down the human nervous system so that the natural resistance to disease and the natural recovery from disease are lowered."

A more comfortable working environment can be achieved by reducing the entry of extraneous noise and by better absorption of indigenous sound. Double glazing will increase the sound insulation value of windows by approximately thirty-five percent and sturdy, well-fitted doors are a further help. Plush carpeting is valuable for the executive office suite, not merely as a status symbol, but because a concrete floor absorbs only one-and-a-half percent of the sound waves which impinge upon it, whereas a carpet absorbs some twenty percent. Even more important are the treatments given to ceilings and walls. The normal range of plaster finishes absorb only two-and-a-half percent of incident sound waves, whereas acoustic tiles absorb from forty to eighty-five percent. Consideration should also be given to silencing the constant ringing of telephones. Ideally, a secretary working in an outside office should screen all but the most essential calls. Telephones are alarm signals. Their abrupt ring inevitably produces a tension response which is sometimes enough to make us jump. In addition they destroy concentration and disrupt a chain of consecutive thought.

Industrial psychologists, in their drive to achieve an egalitarian togetherness, have sometimes advocated lumping together telephonists, typists, clerks, adding machine operators and executives in one large, undivided office precinct. The results have had their psychological fascinations, but operationally they have been disastrous. A group of typists working in a single room generates a noise of more than eighty decibels. This is greater than the noise levels found in busy streets (approximately seventy decibels) and more than enough to reduce the efficiency of cerebral work and cause mental and physical strain.

The managerial working environment needs to be carefully controlled to achieve maximum efficiency with minimum strain. An executive cannot be expected to produce his best work in conditions which are too cold, too hot, smoke-filled or stuffy. In excess heat he becomes lethargic; when the temperature drops too low he is bound to concentrate less on his work and more on the immediate need to keep warm. The ideal temperature for sedentary mental work is somewhere in the region of 68° to 70° F., and it is surely not without significance in this respect that all the major civilizations of the past—Egypt, Persia, East China, Babylon, Carthage, Mexico, Sumeria—have flowered in maritime countries with a mean average temperature of 70°. The ideal climate, in addition to affording an equable temperature, should also provide a comfortable level of humidity. For the executive office suite this should lie somewhere in the region of forty to fifty percent. Humidity levels which are considerably in excess of this tend to induce lethargy. Lower levels, which often arise during the winter when windows are closed and the air dehumidified by excessive heating, produce increased irritability. This was first noticed by a British physician, Dr. E. G. Dexter, who at the turn of the century made a detailed study of the behavior of people in schools, prisons and banks. He found that low levels of humidity were associated with "excessive restlessness of mind." Nervous tension, insomnia and "peculiarities of conduct." The humidity in the arid Sahara desert rarely drops below twenty to twenty-five percent, but in some overheated office suites in the winter it can fall as low as three to five percent! To correct this, containers of water should be placed in front of radiators and heaters, or better still a humidifier installed so that moisture is automatically released into the atmosphere whenever the humidity in the room falls below a certain predetermined level.

Another potential ill effect of working in centrally heated offices is an alteration in the ionization of the air. Normally the atmosphere around us contains millions of electrically charged particles, or ions, which have a stimulating effect on the activity of the body. Unfortunately the polluted air of cities, and the dry, warm air of enclosed offices, frequently shows a depletion of these energizing particles. As a result we tend to feel irritable, stuffy, and prone to headaches. As Dr. Albert Krueger, Professor of Bacteriology at the University of California, says, "People traveling to work in polluted air, spending hours a day in offices or factories, and living their leisure hours in urban dwellings, inescapably breathe ion-depleted air for substantial portions of their lives. There is increasing evidence that this ion depletion leads to discomfort, enervation and lassitude, and loss of mental and physical efficiency." To compensate for this we should open the windows whenever possible or install a machine known as a negative-ion generator which, when plugged into the main electricity circuit, will recharge the atmosphere with invigorating ions.

Even the decor of the executive office suite needs to be chosen with care. Rooms can be soothing or garish, depending on the colors in which they are painted. Experiments show that red excites the nervous system, increases the blood pressure and stimulates the activity of heart and lungs, while colors at the blue end of the spectrum have the opposite effect. Red colors will cheer us up and enliven us; blue colors calm us down. It is inadvisable to use an excess of either of these colors, for an entirely red room would soon prove excessively stimulating, while a totally blue room would give everyone in it a dose of the "blues." The ideal is to achieve a subtle blend of coloring. Work among youngsters in Germany shows that children prefer color-coordinated rooms of predominantly light blue, yellow, yellow-green and orange. In these rooms they are more alert, lively and creative than in rooms painted in what they consider are the ugly colors of white, brown and black. When they were moved to color-coordinated rooms their performance in IQ tests rose by an average of twelve points. When they switched to drab surroundings their ratings fell by an average of fourteen points. It is likely that parallel results would be obtained if similar tests were carried out with executives. We function best, and are most at ease, in quiet, cool, aesthetically designed, harmoniously colored working environments. It is a big mistake to skimp on the design and planning of executive office suites. Some years ago, an architectural journal pointed out that with office building costs amortized over thirty years, the initial capital costs of building represent only two percent of the annual expenses, against routine running costs at six percent and staff salaries at ninety-two percent. The small additional outlay necessary to provide a more comfortable working environment for executives would only marginally increase a company's annual costs, but could produce a large improvement in managerial efficiency. This is particularly true if proper allowance is made for individual idiosyncrasy. No two people agree about what constitutes the ideal working environment. When tests were made to determine the optimum temperature for carrying out heavy work in winter it was found that somebody was comfortable or uncomfortable at every point on the thermometer from 54° to 76° F. A similar divergence of opinion governed the choice of ideal lighting conditions, with sixty-five percent of people opting for a level of illumination ranging anywhere between ten and thirty footcandles. The others requested intensities of lighting which were often considerably above or below this range.

The ideal is to provide environmental conditions which can be altered to suit this wide range of individual preference and to introduce the much-needed stimulus of variety and change. Making such provision will also show we care, and this, as the Hawthorne experiment showed, may be more important than the actual physical changes themselves. As J. C. Brown says in *The Social Psychology of Industry*, "Human beings, whether individually or collectively, react with greater sensitivity to changes in psychological atmosphere, to intentions, implications and suggestions, than they do to any of the ordinary changes in physical environment."

16

SOUNDING THE RETREAT

Everyone has his breaking point if subjected to incessant stress. Experience shows that the most stoical characters will break down and sign spurious "confessions" if subjected to prolonged brainwashing, and even the hardiest soldiers will show signs of battle fatigue if kept for too long at the front line. The same applies to executives. It is admirable to enter the heat of life's battles, but folly to remain there so long that we are reduced to a state of nervous exhaustion. We become shell-shocked if we do not enjoy the occasional recuperative retreat. The samurai warriors recognized this when they retired from the battlefield to meditate, paint or write poetry. This sensible tradition still persists in Japan where activities such as moon watching, bonsai tree cultivation and ikebana flower arranging are encouraged because they are *furyu*, which means that they provide a peaceful retreat from the agitations of daily life. In the West an executive who took an afternoon off to paint flowers, bird watch or crochet would be thought either effeminate, effete or indolent. Yet this might be the most effective way he could utilize his time.

It is necessary to step back from the fray occasionally in order to regroup our forces and prepare for the next advance. This technique is unfamiliar to many Western businessmen who are trained from childhood onward to tackle every problem head on, by a process of all-out frontal assault. The introduction of a little oriental calm and detachment would often improve things. The Town Council in Teignmouth, Devon, England, suffered many explosive arguments during their council meetings. Then during the thick of one particularly angry debate a councillor collapsed with a heart attack. A colleague said, "I was so fed up with listening to these endless rows that I decided to do something about it." With the sanction of his colleagues he introduced the idea of reading poetry during the Council meetings. This has helped to take the tension out of the debates and induce a spirit of quiet reasonableness. After all, there is rarely one correct method of tackling any particular problem. Conflict is caused when committee members stubbornly insist that things must always be done their way. Allowing the other party to do things their way is often the best solution for all concerned. And, as many wives have found, the person who backs down on minor points is often more likely to get her own way on major issues. This is one of the techniques for reducing interpersonal stress recommended by the Association for Mental Health. "Give in occasionally," they suggest.

The wily fighter is not always on the attack. He learns the advantage of rolling with the punches and taking the occasional breather leaning against the ropes.

Two Cornell psychologists studied the effect of stress on a flock of sheep. They subjected certain of the sheep to a series of mild electric shocks. This they found had no visible effect on their behavior. So they introduced an additional element of stress. Ten seconds before the shocks were given they rang a warning bell. This made the sheep apprehensive, to the extent that whenever the bell rang they stopped what they were doing and waited anxiously for the shock to arrive. Once they had received it they resumed their normal activities and carried on as if nothing had happened. It was discovered, however, that if this apprehensive stress was constantly repeated the sheep showed signs of nervous fatigue—they quit eating, stopped following the rest of the flock, lay down dejectedly, and finally showed signs of distressed breathing. At that point the experiments were stopped or the sheep would have died. Subsequent studies showed that these symptoms of nervous breakdown could be prevented if the sheep were given a minimum of two hours' respite from stress in every twenty-four hours. This was just sufficient to enable their nervous systems to recover from the battering they had received in the preceding hours.

It can be a mistake to extrapolate from results gained in animal experiments, but in this case there is ample evidence to confirm that man's behavorial response to stress is very similar to that of the Cornell sheep. Instinctively we protect ourselves from strain by taking the occasional recuperative break.

A team of German physiologists carried out a detailed study of the work pattern of a large group of factory workers in Dortmund and found that the men took rest breaks whenever they were physiologically required, but hid them from their supervisors by indulging in a range of time-wasting activities such as idly polishing their machines. In one factory it was discovered that as much as eleven percent of the day was spent in these unauthorized breaks. In order to maximize the benefit of these idle periods it was decided to introduce official rest breaks of five minutes at the end of every hour. When this was done the hidden breaks disappeared, fatigue was lessened and production, instead of falling, rose by thirteen percent. Similar results have been obtained in many other factories, particularly those in Communist countries. But as yet it is impossible to lay down any hard and fast rules about the optimum timing or length of these breaks. No doubt this varies with the nature of the job. The ideal is to pause before mental fatigue sets in and efficiency wanes. Once this point is reached the body will, in any case, insist on taking a rest. That is the time when our brains go on the blink and our minds, instead of concentrating on the task in hand, escape into flights of recuperative daydreaming. Far better, surely, to take a controlled break when we need it, rather than wait until mental lapses occur.

One of the most valuable times to take a rest is immediately after lunch, when blood is shunted from the brain to the actively working digestive organs. At this time we inevitably experience a degree of "post-prandial torpor." A number of executive offices now boast a relaxation couch or reclining cat-nap chair where quick naps can be taken. Victor Gollancz, the crusading British publisher, used to take a quick snooze on his office couch every afternoon and gave orders that he was not to be disturbed during this time. He found these few moments after lunch an invaluable source of relaxation and refreshment. Tests on college students show that people who find time to take a decent afternoon nap feel less anxious afterwards, are more energetic, and show a fifteen percent increase in the speed of their reactions.

But then there is no reason why cat naps should be limited to the early afternoon. Rests can equally well be taken at other periods of the day. Most animals when left to their own devices take their sleep at irregular intervals during the day. When they are tired they automatically take a short nap and wake refreshed and reinvigorated. Only custom limits our sleep to the hours of darkness. If we followed our natural inclination and took a brief nap whenever we felt tired we would suffer far less nervous strain. This has been the secret of many famous men. Winston Churchill slept whenever he felt the need. When conferences at the White House reached the point of seeming deadlock, President Kennedy would call a halt and while others smoked or drank he would rest his head on the desk and sleep. President Lyndon Johnson insisted on an afternoon nap "with my britches off," President Ford developed to a fine art the habit of sleeping on plane and car trips, while the inventor Thomas Edison would work long, irregular hours in his laboratory and when he was tired snatch three or four hours' sleep on a couch and then return refreshed to his work. But possibly the most imperturbable catnapper of all was the Duke of Wellington, who was found during the height of the Battle of Waterloo dozing behind a copy of the London *Sun*. All these men discovered for themselves the value of making the occasional strategical retreat from life's hurly burly.

A good night's sleep is a further help in this respect. "Sleep," in Shakespeare's words, "that knits up the ravell'd sleave of care, . . . sore labour's bath, balm of hurt minds, great nature's second course, chief nourisher in life's feast." Most of us do not partake enough of this natural restorative. A study of a group of Canadians showed that people who get less than seven hours' sleep a night are more prone to suffer anxiety, tension and fatigue than those who normally sleep longer. When these "sleep-cheats" were encouraged to get an extra couple of hours' rest a night for a month they unanimously reported that at the end of the period they felt better, suffered less tension, anxiety and fatigue, and were better able to cope with stress.

Equally valuable are the days, weekends or longer spells of relaxation. As Dr. Beric Wright, medical adviser to England's Institute of Directors, says, "A holiday is probably the most valuable insurance policy of all against stress, disease and fatigue." What a little medical research has been done on the subject suggests that many executives are taking holidays that are not wholly appropriate to their needs. Professor Pierre Delbarre, Dean of the Faculty of Medicine at the Cochin Port Royal Hospital, Paris, suggests that we should be taking more frequent breaks. "Biological imperatives," he suggests, demand that we should take two or three periods of eight to ten days' vacation a year since this helps prevent the buildup of tension and fatigue. He also recommends that holidays should be taken in the spring and autumn when we are most likely to feel fatigued, rather than in the height of the summer when our metabolism and ability to work are at a peak. We should also pay more attention to correcting the "biological disequilibria" of our lives, he advises, and less to acquiring a tan or rushing off to visit faraway places. Those whose lives consist of endless overseas business trips might find it better to take a leisurely holiday at home. Those who work in the city should enjoy the peace of the countryside, those whose lives are boring should seek excitement, those whose jobs are noncreative should spend their leisure time painting, sculpting, writing or woodworking. In this way we restore a healthy physical and mental balance and make even a short holiday a period of genuine *re-creation*.

17
LEARNING TO SWITCH OFF

To succeed in business an executive needs to be "switched on." To survive its emotional pressures and heavy work demands he needs to acquire the equally essential art of "switching off."

This can be done with the aid of drugs. Throughout the ages man has sought pharmacological relief from stress. South African Indians found a temporary escape from their problems by chewing the dried leaves of the coca plant, which is a rich source of cocaine. Chinese coolies obtained their instant nirvana by smoking a pipe of opium, Arab fellaheen by drawing on hashish-filled hookahs, and Siberian peasants by chewing sub-lethal doses of the "sacred" mushroom. This was the herbal path to happiness and the simplest way for them to ensure a brief respite from life's trials and tribulations. Today the same effect is obtained by taking psychotropic drugs. We have entered the Brave New World where pills can provide cheerfulness when we are sad, tranquility when we are agitated, sleep when we are inappropriately alert, and wakefulness when we are pathologically fatigued. This widespread mood manipulation is not without its risks. As Sir Derrick Dunlop, Chairman of the British Safety of Drugs Committee, says, "There is no such thing as a completely safe and effective medicine."

One of the major drawbacks of taking tranquilizers is that they are totally nonspecific in their action. They may filter off stress, but at the same time they suppress all the other stimuli upon which our safety and effectiveness depends. It is as if a motorist took to wearing a blindfold at night to avoid the glare of approaching headlamps.

Tranquilizers lessen an animal's natural dominance and help to undermine an executive's mien of authority. They can also reduce his effectiveness in other ways. Workers at Washington University, St. Louis, have found that taking Valium lowers concentration and leads to a reduction in reading speeds. It also hampers manual skills, and by slowing reaction times, can lead to an increased risk of road accidents.

More important still is the effect of chemical tranquilization on group behavior. Doctors at the Psychopharmacology Laboratory at Harvard Medical School tested the action of Librium on people working together and found that this commonly prescribed tranquilizer can increase, rather than decrease, hostility. The group were given a task to do and then were told that because they had performed it inadequately they would have to do it again. At this point the people taking tranquilizers showed more aggression than those taking none. The Harvard research team concluded that taking Librium can lead to an increase in aggression, which may appear only when people are involved in frustrating or stressful interpersonal relationships. Doctors refer to this as the "paradoxical" action of tranquilizers. Many cases of child abuse are now attributed to this phenomenon. Mothers may give vent to their pent-up aggression when tranquilizers loosen their inhibitions. In this way the effect of tranquilizers is very similar to that of alcohol. Take a couple of large brandies and go to bed, and you will sleep like a lamb. Take the same amount and have an altercation with your wife, and you will roar like a lion.

For these reasons drugs are not a satisfactory long-term solution to the problem of executive stress. Nor is alcohol, that other favorite method of escape. Noah got drunk to celebrate his survival from the flood, and ever since we have been trying to drown our troubles in drink, only to find that they are invariably expert swimmers. Nowadays the consumption of alcohol is firmly established as the Western male's favorite recreational activity. Devotees find it pleasurable, relaxing and convivial. There is also considerable medical evidence to support the old contention that "a little of what you fancy does you good." Recent research shows that moderate doses of alcohol help to improve the circulation of people suffering from arterial disease. Small quantities also stimulate the flow of the digestive juices, thus supporting St. Paul's injunction, "Use a little wine for thy stomach's sake." Tests on motorists show that a single glass of sherry can improve driving performance by lessening tension and anxiety, and a study at the Boston State Hospital revealed that a pint of beer was a more effective therapeutic agent for geriatric patients than their normal psychotropic drug, Thioridazine. What is more, statistical studies show that moderate drinkers live longer than total abstainers. But while the enjoyment of modest quantities of alcohol is beneficial, the consumption of an excess is equally harmful. The evidence suggests that after cancer and heart disease, alcoholism is the United States' biggest health hazard, causing thousands of deaths each year from cirrhosis of the liver, suicide and road accidents.

In industry, alcoholism presents a particular problem, because it lowers efficiency, mars judgment and increases sickness absenteeism. It is far more the boss's disease than heart attacks and peptic ulcers. A survey of the effects of alcoholism in Cambridgeshire, England, showed that alcoholism was practically twice as common among managers as among professional men. This is not surprising. As the doctors carrying out the survey commented, "Competition in business gives rise to tension, anxiety, frustration, which may be relieved by drinking. Apart from this an elaborate lunch or dinner where drink is freely available is part of the 'softening up' process made possible by our present fiscal and social practices. It is easy to understand that businessmen may drift into alcoholism on account of frequent and excessive drinking associated with their work—a situation recognized by the term 'luncheon alcoholic.' "

Prolonged drinking on this scale can produce permanent brain damage. Dr. Melvin Knisely, Professor of Anatomy at the Medical College of South Carolina, has produced evidence which shows that a risk is involved in even "social drinking." A few brain cells are killed, he finds, whenever a person drinks to the point of feeling slightly giddy. After a heavy drinking bout as many as ten thousand brain cells may be permanently damaged or destroyed. To derive the relaxing benefits of drinking without suffering any of its major toxic hazards, it is necessary to keep the consumption of alcohol within sensible limits. Just over a century ago a Scottish physician, Dr. Francis Anstie, laid down the "safety limit" for drinkers as one-and-a-half ounces of fluid alcohol per day. This is equivalent to half a bottle of wine, two pints of beer, or three and a half single measures of whiskey. Subsequent research confirms the soundness of this advice. A short while ago the U.S. Health Department in its report *Alcohol and Health* said: "The classical Anstie's Limit still seems to reflect the safe amount of drinking which does not substantially increase the risk of early death." Ideally, as Anstie recommended, drinks should be taken with meals, and well diluted with either water, soda, fruit juices or tonic. Another precaution is for drinkers to have the occasional break of two or three dry days to give their livers a chance to recuperate.

As yet we have some way to go before we can offer safe chemical tranquilization. There is no pill on the horizon equivalent to the drug Soma, which Aldous Huxley envisaged would be developed to provide us with a safe and simple escape from the world of harsh reality.

Until it arrives, executives are being asked to make do with a range of pacifying placebos and toys. In America the sale of worry beads and calming stones is rising. Mansized sand pits are beginning to appear in New York office suites. Described as "excellent pacifiers," they are designed so that anxious executives can sit on the edge of the box and soothingly run their fingers through the sand. In Oak Brook, Illinois, executives of the MacDonald's hamburger restaurant chain have been provided with a restroom equipped with a gigantic seven hundred-gallon water bed, the nearest they can possibly get in times of stress to a return to the comfort of their mothers' amniotic fluid. Other stores are marketing a variety of doodling devices which can distract the attention of harassed businessmen. Into this category come the swinging ball bearings and the sand-filled plastic cubes, which when inverted like an egg-timer make intricate patterns in the sand. There is now even an "Executive Security Blanket," complete with suede finish and satin binding, which its makers recommend should be held against the cheek as a comforter in times of stress.

A more fundamental approach to the relief of tension is offered by a wide range of relaxation therapies and meditational exercises. These provide a means of switching off which does not reduce alertness or drive, and does not carry any side effects. Most people who faithfully carry out these exercises report an increased feeling of well-being, a greater release of creative energy, and an increased ability to cope with stress and avoid fatigue.

These techniques range from the simple muscle relaxation exercises contained in Jacobson's system of *Progressive Relaxation*, to the autosuggestive methods advocated in Schultz's *Autogenic Training*, the meditational techniques followed by generations of Christian saints, Buddhist monks and Hindu gurus, and the simplified version adopted by disciples of the Maharishi Mahesh Yoga. Though the details may vary the end result of these techniques is the same—the achievement of a state of physical and mental tranquility.

In 1938 Dr. E. Jacobson, an American, published *Progressive Relaxation* in which he described a technique for combating mental and physical tension by a simple process of "letting go" the muscles of the feet, legs, thighs, buttocks, back, shoulders, neck and face. At about the same time in Europe, Dr. J. H. Schultz developed a technique for inducing relaxation by conjuring up pictures of heaviness and warmth. Modifications of these techniques appear in most contemporary systems of relaxation, together with the concepts of concentration and non-striving, which are an integral part of all forms of meditation. By drawing on these diverse sources it is possible to enumerate certain basic principles which are common to all forms of relaxation therapy. These are:

- *Adopt a relaxing posture.* Any position will do providing it can be maintained with maximum comfort and minimum strain. There are as many positions advocated for practicing relaxation as there are for making love.

  Schultz suggested the "Coachman posture" (seated in a chair with the head and body slumped forward and the forearms resting on the thighs). Yogis recommended the "Lotus" position or the corpse posture (supine, with legs and arms lightly apart from the body). If this latter position (known as the *Shavasana*) causes tension, place a cushion under the knees. This is the relaxing posture advocated for expectant mothers.

- *Enjoy a good stretch.* Just as a yawn prepares the body for sleep, so an overall bodily stretch prepares the body for deeper states of relaxation.

- *Consciously "let go" areas of muscle tension.* Without employing any effort, coax the muscles to relax from toe to tip, paying particular attention to the common sites of muscle tension—the hands, the neck, the jaw, the tongue and the muscles of the face and forehead. If you find this proves difficult, contract the muscles firmly to begin with, and then let them relax. Remember that relaxation is a passive process. It cannot be forced. Just let it happen.

- *Conjure up pictures of heaviness, warmth and relaxation.* Schultz told his patients in a low, soporific voice, "Your arms and hands feel heavy and warm," "Your whole body is peaceful and relaxed," "Warmth is flowing into your feet," "Your feet feel heavy and warm." These hypnotic phrases helped them to relax. Similar feeling can be implanted in the subconscious mind by a process of autosuggestion. It also helps to take fantasy trips into a world of warmth and ease. Imagine you are lying in the South of France bathed in sunshine, feel the hot sand beneath you, listen to the sound of the waves lapping gently in the distance, smell the hibiscus flowers. Or, in your mind's eye, take a stroll through a country meadow, listen to the hum of the bees and the melodious call of the birds, feel the soft touch of the summer breeze upon your cheeks and savor the smell of newmown hay.

Just as anxiety and fear are caused by undisciplined flights of imagination, so can controlled use of mental fantasy induce feelings of peace and repose.

- *Concentrate the mind with the aid of a mental focus.* In order to prevent the intrusion of worrying thoughts concentrate on a relaxing object, activity or phrase. Gaze at a rose, look at an intricate pattern such as the mandala used by Hindu meditators, contemplate your navel or chant a repetitive phrase or religious mantra. The essence of Transcendental Meditation is the repetition of a personal phrase or mantra, which for one pupil was the trisyllabic sound *Shee-Ah-Mah.* This simple technique has been used by some thirty companies in America who claim that it improves job performance, enhances staff relationships, reduces tensions and increases job satisfaction.

Research at the Thorndike Memorial Laboratory, Harvard University, however, shows that the actual words used are immaterial. "A similar technique used with any sound or phrase or prayer or mantra brings forth the same physiologic changes noted during Transcendental Meditation," they find. Many, in fact, will find it more evocative to repeat a meaningful phrase such as "I am at peace with the world" or "I am tranquil, serene and calm."

The concentrative technique favored by the Harvard Research team is to focus during breathing on the flow of air in and out of the nose, slowly repeating the word "one" with every expiration. Inevitably the mind will wander from these chosen focal points. This must be expected, particularly during the early days of meditational practice, and must be checked by returning constantly to the selected focal point.

While relaxing, breathe slowly, deeply and rhythmically. Tension is invariably accompanied by a rapid, shallow pattern of respiration; relaxation by deep ventilation which is more like a heavy sigh than a nervous pant.

Practice these exercises at least once a day for ten to twenty minutes. Ideally this should be done in a quiet environment at a time when there is little danger of interruption. However many people have successfully learned to relax in crowded underground trains, during office coffee breaks, before falling asleep in bed at night or while sitting in the lavatory.

Tension is a habit and so is relaxation. The more we practice either state the more habitual it becomes. Life is fraught with stressful situations, but we can learn to switch off if we want to, and we can do this by learning techniques of relaxation which do not require the use of alcohol or drugs.

18
LETTING OFF STEAM

Things are not always what they seem. As Freud showed, there is often enacted behind the closed curtain of bourgeois respectability a private melodrama of repressed violence, hidden fears and secret longings. Like quiescent volcanoes we maintain an appearance of outward calm while seething like cauldrons within. The denial or repression of these feelings can lead to continual tension and stress. The housewife who constantly tenses her diaphragm to hold back the tears may develop abdominal cramps. The executive who bottles up his rage suffers an increased secretion of acid in his stomach and may develop a gastric ulcer literally through stewing in his own juice. Both would benefit by giving vent to their hidden feelings. Catharsis for them would be good for the soul.

Unfortunately this is an outlet denied to many executives, who feel they must maintain an outward appearance of calm composure whatever they are suffering within. It is all very well for a garage mechanic to rant and rage when things go wrong, or for a messenger boy to hurl obscenities, but the boss must always exude an aura of quiet tranquility. At some point, however, even he may need to let off steam.

The most common way of doing this is by talking it out with a sympathetic colleague. Here again executives may be at a distinct disadvantage, for discretion often decrees that they must keep their worries to themselves. Some, in the relative anonymity of a bar, may pour out their troubles to a kindly barmaid whom tradition equips with a sympathetic smile, a ready ear, a soothing tongue, a broad shoulder to cry on, a large comforting bosom, and a conveniently short memory. Others visit a psychiatrist. Most favored are those executives who can confide in their wives or unload their troubles by talking to a close friend outside the business.

In Japan this simple form of abreaction is offered on a commercial basis. Since 1973 the Tokyo telephone exchange has run a special "Grudge-line" which is open twenty-four hours a day. This enables embittered employees and hen-pecked husbands to listen to a brief message from a sympathetic female voice inviting them to lay bare their souls. After this they can yell, moan, grumble or curse to their heart's content. This service obviously met a very real need, for soon after it was installed an average of fifteen hundred calls a day were being received, making it necessary to extend the facility to embrace a battery of two hundred telephones.

Others feel no need for a sympathetic listener and are quite content to cast their feelings to the wind in a string of well-chosen oaths. They experience relief when they uncork the stopper of polite censorship and give vent to a stream of invective. But executives are rarely given to this form of emotional release. A survey in America showed that factory workers in the Midwest used twenty-four times more swear words than white-collar workers, although even they tripled their use of bad language at parties when alcohol loosened their tongues and they were away from the discipline of their offices. Some psychiatrists advise their patients to swear to get things off their chest. They suggest they curse and scream freely, preferably at times when they are on their own and least likely to be overheard, as when taking a shower or driving a car.

Many societies in their wisdom have provided culturally acceptable ways for people to let off steam. The Greeks had their Dionysian feasts and the Romans their Bacchanalian orgies. The Latin American nations hold regular carnivals, the Germans their annual beer festivals and the Eskimos stage occasional "drumming contests." These contests are colorful events in which feuding rivals indulge in a ritualized slanging match. Egged on by their neighbors, family and friends, they do verbal battle until honor is satisfied, anger dissipated and friendship restored. But tradition in America and Britain abhors the show of violent emotion. Even the outward expression of passion is culturally taboo. From childhood onward we are urged to keep a stiff upper lip. We have no equivalent of the public orgy or festival; only Christmas, Thanksgiving Day and the office party, and these are hardly equally liberating. Yet the more closely integrated the society we live in, the greater its need for emotional release.

When small groups of men are confined together for long periods in a nuclear submarine or on an expedition they frequently show signs of emotional stress which is known to doctors as "polar disease" or "expedition choler." Because of their close dependence on one another the men are loath to fight. So, at great cost to their emotional equilibrium, they bottle up their feelings, swallow their rage and deny their frustration. In this dilemma, says the noted ethologist Konrad Lorenz. "The man of perception finds an outlet by creeping out of the barracks (tent, igloo) and smashing a not too expensive object with as resounding a crash as the occasion merits."

Our varying emotional states are accompanied by physiological changes which prepare the body for whatever action is most suited to the mood. When we are angry our muscles tense; fats and sugars, the fuels of muscular exercise, are poured into our bloodstream; blood pressure rises and our pulse quickens. In this way we are prepared for battle. In case we get injured in the ensuing struggle, the clotting power of our blood is also increased, to help staunch the wounds. If action is taken these physiological changes are utilized and we quickly revert to the emotional and biochemical status quo. But if we decide that a soft answer would be more likely to turn away wrath, or that it would be more diplomatic to smile benignly than to kick an infuriating sales director in the crotch, these physiological changes remain. If persistent they may lead to hypertension and recurrent fibrositic pains. Coronary disease is another possible sequel, since the elevated fat and sugar levels in the blood encourage the formation of atheromatous plaques in the walls of the coronary arteries, while the heightened coagulability of the blood favors the formation of blood clots.

To avoid these unfortunate consequences we should seek an alternative form of action when we cannot directly express our emotions. This is a strategy employed by most animal species. It is described by ethologists as "displacement activity." Herring gulls may threaten each other by lifting their heads and spreading their wings, then instead of fighting retire and expend their energy tearing at the grass. Even more unusual is the displacement activity of the normally belligerent three-spined stickleback. Instead of fighting with their neighbors they will stand on their heads and burrow furiously in the sand. We, often unconsciously, adopt similar techniques. The expectant father paces nervously up and down the corridor outside the maternity ward. Children, instead of beating their parents, will throw a teddy bear across the room. Adults when frustrated chew pencils, slam doors, stamp their feet or kick the cat. All are displacement activities which help to lift the lid off the emotional pressure-cooker.

A mail order firm in Los Angeles has made a specialty of facilitating human displacement activity. It offers a variety of "aggression release equipment," including four-foot dolls which can be viewed as surrogate bosses or parents and roughly treated, and sturdy, foam rubber "Encounter-bats" with which you can safely lambast anyone who annoys you. As the company's founder, Richard Epstein, says: "Psychologists have always encouraged people to give vent to their feelings." One psychiatrist, Dr. Roger Tre-gold, of University College Hospital, London, suggests that every office and factory should have a "violence room" where employees can let off steam by smashing cheap crockery or belaboring punchballs. This principle is employed in Japan, where the giant Matsushita Electrical Industrial Company has constructed a "self-control room" equipped with two life-sized dummies and a generous supply of bamboo staves. Here employees are encouraged to find a vicarious release for their pent-up rage by beating the dummies until their fury is spent.

A similar technique is used by psychologists, particularly followers of the school of "Bio-energetics," who get their frustrated patients to take a tennis racquet or simply use their fists to beat a cushion or bed, screaming out as they do so, "You bitch! I'll kill you!" or other appropriate words. They continue to bellow and rage, urged on by the therapist and other members of the group, until their anger is spent or they dissolve into tears.

While there is an undoubted benefit to be derived from abreaction, there are also certain inherent risks. There is, for example, the very real possibility that the dramatic cathartic games played by encounter groups may at times stimulate aggression rather than release it. This point was entertainingly made by a reader of the *Wisconsin State Journal*. She was distressed that the newspaper's advice column had suggested that the mother of a three-year-old child with temper tantrums should let the child kick the furniture to get the anger out of its system. The dismayed reader wrote a letter to the editor pointing out, "My younger brother used to kick the furniture when he got mad. Mother called it 'letting off steam.' Well, he's thirty-two years old now and still kicking the furniture—what's left of it, that is. He is also kicking his wife, the cat, the kids and anything else that gets in the way. Last October he threw the television set out of the window when his favorite team failed to score and lost the game. (The window was closed at the time.) Why don't you tell mothers that children should be taught to control their anger?"

Both children and adults need to steer a course between emotional repression and undisciplined self-expression. We should not fear aggression, for anger can be constructive as well as destructive, but equally well we should never allow it to get totally out of control. Like dynamite, it is a powerful tool which should be handled "Handle with Care." When properly used it can move mountains, but when irresponsibly employed it can wound and kill.

We become angry when we are frustrated in our attempts to secure our short- or long-term goals. Aggression is the heaven-sent emotive driving force which encourages us to overcome the obstacles in our way. Without it we would capitulate at every reverse and cheerfully settle for a more easily obtainable second best. A successful executive needs plenty of aggressive drive, but since he works with others he needs to keep that drive under careful control. He should develop the art of using his aggression in a non-combative way. This means whenever possible attacking a situation or event rather than a person. His sole aim must be to remove the source of frustration and advance the welfare of the company, not to belittle or wound. When he criticizes his subordinates he should bear in mind the principles outlined in Chapter 8. To tell another person you are angry with him can be therapeutic for both parties. Often it clears the air. Possibly for months he may have misinterpreted the cause of your annoyance, or been totally unaware that he had upset you. To provide him with some feedback gives him the opportunity to modify his behavior. This paves the way to closer understanding and the forging of more satisfactory working relationships. It is possible for colleagues to share their work, travel, time and ideas and yet remain comparative strangers. They become friends only when they share their feelings.

As Jung said, "Real liberation comes not from glossing over or repressing painful states of feeling but only from experiencing them to the full."

19
THE ART OF ACCEPTANCE

We are rarely satisfied with what we have. A businessman wants to increase his income, his wife is anxious to buy some new living-room curtains, their daughter yearns to be more beautiful, their son longs to be a better football player. When we have no car we are keen to get hold of anything on four wheels. Once we have got a five-year old jalopy we are ashamed to park it beside our neighbor's brand new Ford and immediately long for something better. Discontent is built into our systems, encouraged by an advertising industry which is bent on making us dissatisfied with whatever we have. Whatever our current possessions someone will undoubtedly say they are too small, too old, too slow, too commonplace, too drab or too dreadfully outmoded. We buy more in an attempt to purchase a better life, forgetting that the good life exists only when we stop wanting a better one. We need occasionally to step off the relentless treadmill and savor what we have, rather than constantly yearn for what we have not.

This nagging discontent is a common cause of stress. For example, when a study was made of the personalities of a large group of migraine sufferers it was found that they were so preoccupied with their struggle to attain higher goals that they rarely provided themselves with what were described as "resting points of contentment." Like many politicians and religious fanatics, they were so busy building a better tomorrow that they had no time to sit back and enjoy their thoroughly enjoyable today. They were dreaming of tomorrow's *filet mignon* when they should have been enjoying today's pizza.

This is a common human failing. As Abraham Maslow showed, we all have a hierarchy of needs. We set out first of all to satisfy our primitive needs for warmth, food, shelter and sex. Once we have met these basic needs we try to gratify some of our less pressing demands for companionship, excitement and play. Then we demand self-fulfillment and an outlet for our creative talents. When these higher needs are met, we are still not satisfied but set our sights higher still and demand perhaps the aesthetic pleasure of music and art. We show, in fact, what the Christian theologians describe as the *cor irrequietum*—the restless heart. We are constantly seeking something better. But this constant search for betterment must not be allowed to hamper the relaxed enjoyment of what we already possess.

It is easy for managers to feel cheated when their employees fail to appreciate their current level of welfare benefits. Factory workers still find cause for complaint even though they have been given better wages, a five-day week, shorter working hours, pensions, cleaner working conditions, increased job security and enhanced job satisfaction. In the face of this flagrant ingratitude it is easy to advocate a return to a more authoritarian style of management. But this would do no good. People will always seek to improve their lot. According to Maslow, "We should . . . never expect a cessation of complaints; we should expect only that these complaints will get to be higher and higher complaints, i.e. that they will move from the lower-grumble level to higher-grumble levels and finally to metagrumble levels." When an employee stops to complain about the seasoning of the cafeteria soup you can be sure he is not suffering from starvation and is reasonably satisfied with his pay. Nevertheless, if we are to achieve a reasonable level of contentment, we must learn to enjoy "resting points of contentment" in our lives.

We must also have the honesty to accept ourselves as we really are. Denial is one of the subconscious mind's favorite defense mechanisms. We feel shy, but rather than face up to the fact, we compensate by being excessively brash. We lack an education in the arts but nevertheless struggle to maintain the pose of a cultured aesthete. This deception involves a degree of continuing stress, for if we refuse to be ourselves, we must constantly suffer the strain of acting an alien role. One unguarded word or act and the mask can slip. The ability to accept ourselves as we truly are has been described by psychiatrist Dr. Karl Menninger as an "inner strength." Philosopher William James regarded it as the "religion of healthy mindedness."

Further stress arises from our unwillingness to accept the inevitable. Long-distance swimmers know that it is often foolish to try to swim against the tide. Far better to travel with it until the tide turns or you can catch a favorable in-shore current. The same principle applies in everyday life. There is a time to set full sail and forge ahead, and another when it is wiser to lower sails and ride out the storm or even limp back into harbor until the storm abates. To quote Shakespeare, "There is a tide in the affairs of men, which, taken at the flood, leads on to fortune." The wise man seizes his chances, but also bows to the inevitable.

We waste energy and suffer needless stress when we beat our heads against impenetrable walls. The secret is to maintain a degree of flexibility and be prepared to adapt ourselves to our environment, rather than try to modify the environment to meet our preconceived ideas and plans. King Canute was foolish because he attempted to stop the flowing tide. Mohammed, on the other hand, showed his wisdom because he accepted that inevitably he would have to move to the mountain, since the mountain could not possibly move to him.

Faith, we are told, can move mountains, but experience shows that it is generally better to leave the mountain where it is and find a pathway around. In orienteering, a contestant learns that a straight line is not necessarily the shortest distance between two points on a map. Experience enables him to find the quickest way of traversing a cross-country route, and if a swamp, cliff or unfordable stream lies between him and the next checkpoint on the map he immediately picks out an alternative way. He does not waste time attempting the impossible or tackling unnecessary obstacles. Yet every step he takes, even if it is to double back or take a two-minute breather, is planned to bring him closer to his goal.

So it should be in life. There is a great gulf between obduracy, apathy and acceptance. Obduracy often attempts the impossible; apathy gives up without differentiating between what can and cannot be achieved; but acceptance makes the distinction and channels energy into purely practical endeavors. As writer Arthur Gordon puts it, "Apathy paralyzes the will-to-action; acceptance frees it by relieving it of impossible burdens."

Stress is also reduced when we accept with resignation life's inevitable setbacks and misfortunes. William inherited a large sum of money from his father and proceeded to quadruple it by a series of astute business enterprises. Then came the Depression and he was forced into bankruptcy. He could easily have sat back and bemoaned his fate. Instead he fought back. He went on welfare, took a job as a laborer, and earned a little extra cash by carrying out one or two business transactions in his spare time. Throughout the Depression he kept cheerful and hopeful that his fortune would eventually change. Then both he and his wife developed abdominal cancers. Their operations took all his painstakingly acquired savings. He survived the operation, but his beloved wife died. Soon after, he developed cancer of the larynx, but once again was treated and cured. Throughout his adversity he maintained a state of cheerful optimism. As his doctor said: "He still goes around the town, smiling, interested in everything, and interesting everyone in something."

One of his neighbors, amazed that he could stay serene throughout so much misfortune, asked him for his secret. "I'll tell you," he replied. "A long time ago I sat down to try and figure out my next move. I thought a long time. And then the answer came to me. I got up and repeated it to myself, 'William, you might just as well cooperate with the inevitable.' And that's what I've been doing ever since —cooperating with the inevitable."

To avoid stress we need to develop the Spanish philosophy of *Que será, será*.

Stress, like disease, only comes when there is conflict. Hippocrates pointed out that with disease there is not only *pathos* (suffering) but also *ponos* (toil). Many of the outward symptoms of disease—the redness of inflammation, the pallor of shock and the breathlessness of heart failure— are only the outward expression of the body's fight to restore its inward equilibrium. So it is also with stress. If we cease to struggle we do not suffer mental dis-ease. This is a principle practiced by Professor Hans Selye. Whenever he gets keyed up about something, he stops to ask himself whether it is really worth the trouble. Whenever his equanimity is threatened he repeats a little jingle: "Fight always for the highest attainable aim, but never put up resistance in vain." This helps him preserve his nervous energy for tasks which are both practical and important.

To live at peace with ourselves and our environment we need to develop the art of accepting what we have, what we are, what happens and what is. More especially we need the wisdom to know when we should accept these things, and when they can and should be changed. As the old prayer says, "Oh Lord, grant me the strength to change the things that need changing, the courage to accept the things that cannot be changed, and the wisdom to know the difference."

20
THE GIFT OF PLAY

All work and no play makes Jack a dull boy. It also makes him rigid, myopic and tense.

Man's need for work is obvious. His equal need for play is less apparent. In its report *Sports and the Community*, the British Central Council of Recreation's Wolfenden Committee concluded: "Man needs play. In the form of a game, a sport or an outdoor activity of some kind, it is desirable in itself, for its own sake as a valuable element in a full and rounded life." Play helps to bring about a reduction of frustration, tension and stress. It provides opportunities for:

- *Distraction.* Everyday worries fade from view when our attention is focused on play. It is difficult to worry about dwindling overseas sales when you are trying to sink an eighteen-foot putt, or speculate about an impending takeover bid when you are playing a hand of bridge. The mind is never completely at rest. It cannot be turned off, but it can be switched over to another program. Eufemia, one of America's top professional pool players, has taught many executives to improve their game. "Pool," he finds, "is a great brainwasher. You can't play with anything else on your mind." That is true of most other hobbies and sports.

- *Diversion.* According to Dr. Selye, individuals need rest only when they are subject to an excess overall load of stress. At other times, when only one part of their nervous system is overloaded, they need diversion. This is a far more common need. As Pavlov wrote, "If we look through the skull into the brain of a consciously thinking person, and if the place of optimal excitability were luminous, then we should see playing over the cerebral surface a bright spot with fantastic, waving borders, constantly fluctuating in size and form, and surrounded by a darkness, more or less deep, covering the rest of the hemisphere." When we work and worry we risk fatiguing one small part of our mental mechanism. When we play we shift the area of excitation and reduce the risk of local overstimulation. A change like this is often as good as a rest.

- *Abreaction.* Play enables us to let off steam and escape from the disciplines and routines of our working life. Inside every adult there is a playful child struggling to escape. A child who longs perhaps to play with toy soldiers or an electric train set, but feels too inhibited to do so. We are trained to think that adults should shun childish pleasures and always show a staid and dignified front. But politicians, judges and company directors need to let their hair down occasionally and kick a football in the garden, frolic in the hay, or romp with the dogs in the park. This helps them lose their inhibitions and escape from the constant seriousness of their work. A German psychiatrist, Tobias Brocher, head of the sociopsychology department of Frankfurt's Sigmund Freud Institute, has set up a "play school for parents" in the small town of Ulm. His experience shows that adults can sometimes lose their hangups and infantile repressions by indulging in childlike play. One stern, inflexible judge learned to relax through finger-painting. To begin with he would only unbend enough to dip his finger into a pot of white paint and make a formal pattern of orderly dots. Three weeks later he had overcome his inhibitions and was able to wallow in paint up to his elbows and plaster the walls with splashes of vivid red, yellows and browns. "Isn't it fun?" Brocher asked him. With a shy grin the judge admitted, "I was never permitted as a child to play with mud; my mother punished me when I came home dirty." Now at last he was able to discover the fun he had missed as a child.

We can escape the stresses of work if during our leisure hours we allow the child inside us to escape and indulge in uninhibited play.

- *Freedom*. In moments of play we break free from the routine of our everyday life. We leave behind the discipline of work and temporarily escape the frustrating rules and conventions which society imposes upon us. We are at liberty to daydream, to invent our own regulations, to do our own thing. As Sartre has said, "As soon as man apprehends

himself as free and wishes to use his freedom . . .
then his activity is play."

- *Self-expression.* Play provides an opportunity for
  exercising those facets of our personality which
  cannot find expressions within the confines of our
  work. It is noticeable that the inmates of political
  prison camps and penal institutions frequently use
  games and hobbies as a way of reaffirming their
  individuality. In many ways men who give themselves entirely to their work become as rigidly
  institutionalized as long-term prisoners. They take
  on the persona of the organization for which they
  work, and when retirement forces them to sever the
  firm's umbilical cord they are as lost as long-term
  prisoners released into the outside world after years
  in jail.

  Play provides a safe arena within which we can
  develop our capabilities. Machiavellian cunning
  can be fostered playing poker, stamina increased by
  rock-climbing, linguistic skills honed by completing
  crossword puzzles and deductive powers enhanced
  by playing chess. We improve our ability to work
  in a team by playing football, increase our patience
  by going fishing, our powers of observation by bird-
  watching and our speed and accuracy of judgment
  by competing in motor rallies. Through play we
  develop new skills, explore fresh ground and overcome old fears and fantasies. That is why psychiatrists at Farleigh Hospital, Bristol, England, have
  built an indoor adventure playground "to stimulate
  patients to explore their potential."

- *Learning.* We learn by playing. This is obvious in
  the play activities of children. Girls prepare for

their eventual role as mothers by playing with dolls; boys test out their ability to survive in an aggressively competitive world by wrestling, fighting or striving to run faster or jump higher than their friends.

Ethologists suggest play is a means of learning for all animals. Experiments with chimpanzees show that it is easier to solve a problem if the objects involved have formed the subject of previous play. Hans Haas tells the story of a chimpanzee's attempt to drag a banana into its cage with the aid of two short canes. He tried first using one stick and then the other and finally abandoned the task in a fit of rage. Later, while playing with the sticks, he found he could insert the end of one cane inside the other to form a long, jointed rod. Armed with this discovery he immediately returned to his unresolved task and with the extra length provided by the united canes managed to hook the banana inside the cage. As Hass observed, "Having failed to solve the problem under instinctive pressure he had solved it in the relaxed zone of play. The same must apply to many human discoveries and inventions." As he concluded after reviewing the play activities of animals and man, "Our play and curiosity impulse is responsible not only for discovery, exploration and innovation, but also in large measure, for promoting our artistic development."

- *Relief from anxiety.* Excitement and tension may be generated when we play, but the moment the playing ceases we experience a reduction of tension and anxiety. As the historian Johan Huizinga says in his classic study of human play, *Homo Ludens*: "A feeling of exaltation and tension accompanies the action, mirth and relaxation follow."

Experiments with animals confirm that pleasurable stimulation helps to decrease anxiety. Pleasure centers have been identified in a part of the brain known as the limbic area. If this center is stimulated while laboratory rats are given electric shocks they no longer show their normal anxiety response. A similar mechanism almost certainly operates in man, and one very practical way of lessening the impact of recurrent tensions and anxieties is to indulge in pleasurable play.

It seems to matter little what form of recreation we choose providing it is enjoyable, affords a change from our normal routine, and meets our need for free self-expression. Organized games, though valuable, are in many ways too formal, too rigid and too repetitive to meet our play needs in full. The set-piece Battle of Waterloo may have been won on the playing fields of Eton, but the unpredictable battle of life is more likely to be won by free, unstructured play. When a group of adults were asked what they would most like to do in their leisure time they gave as their favored activities skin diving, sailing, skiing, and horseback riding. These, it is interesting to note, are largely noncompetitive activities containing nonstructured play—ideal recreational pursuits for people coping with the pressures of a stressful, routine working life.

To gain the full benefit of play we must be prepared to be totally uninhibited in its pursuit. We must act spontaneously without bothering what the neighbors will think. The aim is to be childlike without being childish. In this way we give expression to our self-assured maturity, for as the German writer Johann Schiller said, "Man only plays when in the full meaning of the word he is a man, and he is only completely a man when he plays."

It is unlikely that American Presidents will ever feel sufficiently liberated that they will perform cartwheels in public to celebrate their inauguration, or British premiers bathe naked in the fountains at Trafalgar Square. Tradition requires them to adopt a more decorous form of play. Each British premier has had his favorite recreational pursuit. Edward Heath sailed, Churchill painted, Macmillan went grouse shooting; Wilson, Balfour, Asquith, Lloyd George and Ramsay MacDonald played golf, and Chamberlain and Douglas-Home fished. This latter activity seems to be a favorite form of escape for men in high executive office. Herbert Hoover, President during the difficult days of the great Depression, said, "Presidents have only two moments of personal seclusion. One is prayer; the other is fishing—and they cannot pray all the time." The pace of life is immediately slowed when a man goes fishing. In fact the four thousand-year-old inscription on an Assyrian tablet says, "The gods do not subtract from the allotted span of men's lives the hours spent in fishing."

Ideally the relaxed attitude we adopt during moments of play should be allowed to flow into our everyday life. When Plato asked himself the rhetorical question "What is the right way of living?" he gave as his reply: "Life must be lived as play." We should always endeavor to see life's funny side and refuse to take either our work or ourselves too seriously. Laughter is a safety valve, and one of the few ways of letting off steam wholly approved by society. As one psychiatrist observed, "I've seldom been called upon to help a person who had a sense of the ridiculous, and I've *never* had to treat anyone who could really laugh at himself."

In France, Dr. Vachet of the Paris Institute of Psychology encourages students to dispel their tensions and dissolve their anxieties by indulging in uninhibited, rollicking laughter. A similar technique was employed by Abraham Lincoln, who during the height of the Civil War tried to relax the members of his War Cabinet by reading a humorous sketch. But his ministers found it difficult to unwind. "Why don't you laugh?" said the disappointed President. "With the fearful strain that is upon me night and day if I did not laugh I should die, and you need the medicine as much as me."

Laughter is a powerful medicine for people under stress, a safer way of relieving anxiety than taking tranquilizers, and a cheaper form of escape than a prolonged Bermuda vacation. The man who throws custard pies is unlikely to throw temper tantrums, and the person who belly laughs rarely belly aches.

The playful approach to life, as well as lessening tension, also helps increase the quality of our lives. Psychiatrist Erik Erikson made a detailed study of a large group of children. Thirty years later when they had grown into adults he examined them again, and found that the ones leading the most interesting, fulfilling lives were those who had managed to retain a sense of playfulness at the center of their lives.

21
BACK TO NATURE

Man is by nature a pastoral animal. Despite several centuries of industrialization he is still not adapted to the city's crowded clangor. It took the fringe-toed lizard thousands of years to adapt to life in the Arizona desert—to develop webbed feet built like snow shoes to prevent their sinking into the soft ground, nostrils which swing shut like trap doors to keep out the drifting sand, and eyelids which intermesh like zippers to protect the eyes when sandstorms blow. Man's full adaptation to the peculiar demands of contemporary life will also take millennia to achieve. The process of urbanization has occurred too rapidly for our mental well-being. At the beginning of the nineteenth century four-fifths of the British population lived in the country. Then the great urban migration began and by the end of the century only one out of every five lived in rural districts. The new urbanites gained prosperity, but were dispossessed of their traditional work, customs and roots.

During the twentieth century life has become increasingly complex and artificial. Inhabitants of a modern city block, like Chicago's one-hundred-story John Hancock Building, need never leave their concrete pen to battle with the elements. Everything required for their daily existence—department stores, restaurants, banks and cocktail bars—is included within the apartment complex. Montreal has its underground city, the vast Place Ville Marie with its dozen subterranean cinemas and theaters, 330 shops, and 64 restaurants, snack bars and cafés. Here, far removed from green fields, bird song and natural sunlight, it is possible to work and play in a totally controlled environment. America is even developing underground schools, which their advocates say are easier to clean and have the additional advantage of screening the children from outside distractions. Now more than ever youngsters will have to rely on biology textbooks to learn about the birds and bees.

Undoubtedly we will survive in these inimical conditions. Humans are extremely tolerant animals and are known to put up with a level of noise, dirt, discomfort, frustration and misery that would be intolerable for a rabbit or mouse. In fact in many ways we are *too* tolerant for our own good. As Professor René Dubos says in *Man Adapting*, "Life in the modern city has become a symbol of the fact that man can become adapted to starless skies, treeless avenues, shapeless buildings, tasteless bread, joyless celebrations, spiritless pleasures." But we pay a price for this easy acceptance.

It is likely that much of to-day's mental stress arises because we are as yet ill-adapted to an industrial way of life.

Zoologists have noted that the health of animals frequently deteriorates when they are moved from a natural environment and placed in captivity. Autopsies show that the frequency of arteriosclerosis among mammals and birds at the Philadelphia Zoo has increased ten- to twentyfold in the last forty years. This is attributed to the "social pressures" resulting from overcrowding, loss of territory, and the general restriction of activities. Social rivals cannot escape from one another when they are in captivity. After a fight they still have to see each other and this can lead to perpetual conflict. Similar stresses occur in man and in the *Human Zoo* ethologist Desmond Morris suggests that it is more realistic to compare the behavior of man with that of other caged animals. In their natural habitat wild animals do not mutilate themselves, murder, suffer stomach ulcers, become obese, develop arteriosclerosis or form homosexual pair-bonds. In captivity they do all of these things. So does contemporary man in his concrete zoo. As Morris says, "The modern human animal is no longer living in conditions natural for his species. Trapped, not by a zoo collector, but by his own brainy brilliance, he has set himself up in a huge, restless menagerie where he is in constant danger of cracking under the strain."

To alleviate this strain we long to return to the simplicity of the arcadian life. Much of this yearning is at a purely subconscious level. Town dwellers seek to reestablish their links with nature by keeping parrots and tropical fish, growing exotic indoor plants and cultivating town gardens and window boxes. On the weekend there is a mass migration of city dwellers into the great outdoors, where they hike, picnic, sightsee and visit zoos, wildlife parks and nature reserves. Those who can afford it buy a house in the country. (By 1971 twenty percent of urban households in America and Sweden had a second home in the country, but only one percent in England.) For five days of the week an executive will struggle to keep his family in the material comforts of the city, then on the weekend he escapes into the country to rediscover his grass roots and practice the primitive arts and crafts of human survival—chopping wood, making fires, mending broken fences and mowing overgrown grass. The wealthy will now pay a king's ransom to hunt, shoot and fish—activities which once were the necessary chores of survival in peasant communities. Middle-class wives, tired of the monotony of synthetic convenience foods, are returning to baking their own bread from whole wheat, stone-ground flour. In their spare time they weave, throw pots and make home-made wine.

This atavistic trek is probably most noticeable in the young, who are less attracted by convention and more willing to throw overboard the accretions of two centuries of urbanization. Not for them the regimentation, the military hair cuts, stiff collars and ties and formal suits. They are happy to go vegetarian, experiment with macrobiotic food or eat only compost-grown vegetables and fruit. They are prepared for a while at least to dress simply, to live in self-supporting communes and to have few material possessions other than a shirt, a pair of jeans and a sleeping bag.

Enlightened civic planners are also playing their part by preserving city parks, creating garden cities, and planting protective green belts around existing industrial towns. So too are architects, like Finland's Alvar Aalto, who blended structures into their natural environments. He used curved structural beams to reflect the sun's rays and give diffuse natural lighting in museums, and designed buildings to incorporate natural outcrops of rock rather than insisting that the site should first be dynamited. One of

Aalto's guiding principles was that man must remain in closer contact with nature.

This may for him have been chiefly an aesthetic consideration, but it is equally well a sound psychoprophylactic principle. Doctors have reported what appears to be a close causal link between town dwelling and symptoms of psychosocial distress. The prevalence of crime, divorce, desertion, mental breakdown and suicide is higher in towns than in the country, and is particularly high in large, rapidly expanding industrial cities. To escape this source of stress we need occasionally to regress to a simpler, pastoral way of life. People spending weekends in the countryside give a number of reasons for their love of the great outdoors. Some go to revel in the scenery, others to enjoy a break from routine and convention, to live for a while at a slower pace, to exchange artificial values for real values, to recharge batteries, to have a few moments' peace and quiet, or to escape from difficult or demanding human relationships. A closer examination suggests that an occasional return to nature confers six main benefits:

- *It establishes a healthy sense of perspective.* When we contemplate the vastness of the universe it is difficult to have an exaggerated sense of one's own importance. It is humbling to discover that even if every one of the world's three billion inhabitants were six feet tall and a foot-and-a-half wide they could still be packed together in a box no bigger than a half-mile square, pushed over the top of the Grand Canyon and totally lost from sight.

    We are often dazzled by our technological genius, by our ability to create massive generators and nuclear reactors, and yet the motive power of industry is a puny thing compared with the tremendous forces liberated by earthquakes, tempests and electrical storms. In one minute, for example, an average hurricane expends more energy than the United States consumes in half a century.

Faced with these awe-inspiring statistics our day-to-day anxieties seem trivial. They may loom large to us today, but tomorrow they will fade from sight and in a year they will probably be completely forgotten. Compared with the infinite world of nature we and our petty problems are but grains of sand.

- *It induces a feeling of timelessness.* Observation of the world around us should inspire a spirit of patience and calm. We are slaves to haste, but nature refuses to be hurried. Nothing can speed the sunrise, nothing can hasten the rhythm of the tides or the annual rebirth of the flowers. We alone have introduced rush and bustle into the world. We no longer allow things to happen at the leisurely pace at which trees grow, rivers flow and seasons change. Everything has to happen in the shortest possible time and tomorrow it must be quicker still. But when we study the world of nature we are less inclined to stick to rigid deadlines and more willing to let things develop in the fullness of time.

- *It creates a sense of permanence.* When society is in a state of constant flux it is comforting to be reassured of the permanence of the world around us. Mother earth makes up for the vagaries and wild eccentricities of man by being simple, solid, sane and utterly dependable. *Terra firma* has become our hallmark of everything solid and secure. Simple things are described as being "down to earth," and the return to sanity after a period of madness a "coming back to earth." We feel secure when we have our feet firmly planted on the ground, particularly if it happens to be our native land or our own backyard. As Anthony Trollope said, "It is a very comfortable thing to stand on your own ground. Land is about the only thing that can't fly away."

- *It encourages a spirit of quiet meditation.* Most great men have drawn strength and inspiration through communion with nature. As the Psalmist said, "I will lift up mine eyes unto the hills from whence cometh my strength." Generations later Roman citizens climbed the Janicus mountain to seek inspiration. John the Baptist went out into the wilderness to contemplate, and the prophet Mohammed climbed Mount Hira to meditate.

  Conrad Russell, when looking back on the life of his father Bertrand Russell, Nobel-prize winning philosopher, scientist and author, remembers his lifelong communion with nature. He loved the sea and hills. "I remember him, at ninety-five, swinging over the steps of the balcony at Plas Penrhyn for the sheer deilght of the view of Snowdon in the afternoon sun. Above all, I remember him spending hours watching the movement of water in waterfalls. One of my earliest memories is of watching him standing under a waterfall in California, and one of my latest is of him gazing rapt at the fall of water through the rapids of Aberglaslyn in North Wales." And his favorite proverb was "Men of wisdom love the sea; men of virtue love the mountains."

In today's frenetic world men of sanity love nature in all its myriad forms.

- *It engenders a feeling of unity and harmony.* In the process of civilization man has become increasingly divorced from his pastoral setting. An unhealthy schism has developed between man and the world he inhabits. This is seen by theologians as a spiritual disaster. As Cardinal Newman says, "The human race is implicated in some terrible aboriginal calamity. It is out of joint with the purpose of its Creator." To psychologists the rift is regarded more prosaically as a common cause of alienation and distress. As writer Charles Reich says, "Man was uprooted from his supporting physical and social environment and, like a polar bear in a city zoo, he would from then on suffer an alienated existence." When we return to the world of nature we heal the rift and end this unnatural alienation. This relieves the underlying tension and can be a source of unparalleled delight. This is the basis of the mystical experience, those rare moments of ecstasy when time stands still and we seem to be at one with the universe—a condition variously described as "cosmic consciousness," "the transcendental experience" or by Freud as the "oceanic feeling." These moments rarely come when we are engaged in conscious thought, but when we are relaxing and at peace with the world. The writer John Buchan tells in his autobiography of one such experience. It happened when he took an early morning dip and then basked contentedly in the sunshine while his breakfast cooked. Suddenly, he recalls, "scents, sights and sounds blended into a harmony so perfect that it transcended human expression, even human thought. It was like a glimpse of the peace of eternity." Feelings like that may be encountered sitting quietly beside a mountain stream, or lying in a flower-strewn meadow, but they are rarely experienced in night clubs, casinos, dance halls or restaurants.

- *It simplifies life.* Our way of life has become increasingly complicated. We would find it difficult to imagine life today without cars and centrally heated homes. But cars bring traffic jams, breakdowns and parking problems, and homes mean mortgages, repairs and utility bills. The more we need the more we have to worry about. The poor man has no cause to worry about stock market plunges, or tax increases. We worry less if we take the wider, cosmic view and realize that we can flourish with a fraction of what we have today. After all our forebears managed without sugar until the thirteenth century, without buttered bread until the sixteenth century, without soap until the seventeenth, gas and electricity until the nineteenth and cars, canned food and airplanes until the twentieth.

Some people will rediscover their grass roots by going for long country walks. Others will fish, watch birds, grow orchids or study geology. Camping is another pastime that meets this primeval need. It is an activity which gives city dwellers an opportunity to escape from their time-obsessed lives and have the freedom to camp when and where they wish, eat when they will, dress as casually as they please and enjoy the soothing sight of green grass and the soft smells and sounds of the countryside. Charles Lindbergh, writing nearly half a century after he made his solo cross-Atlantic flight, said, "Man must feel the earth to know himself and recognize his values." He himself made this contact by going on regular camping trips. "The great difference between a tent and a house," he wrote, "is that a tent introduces you to the earth, while a house separates you from it. . . . In a sleeping-bag, after an ember-cooked meal, you feel free of civilization's elaborate accoutrements and realize the basic simplicity of life. The only essentials are a covering for your body, a shelter from the weather and a little food."

Gardening is another favored retreat. Author Alicia Bay Laurel in her book *Living on the Earth* gives this recipe for relaxation: "Find a little bit of land somewhere and plant a carrot seed. Now sit down and watch it grow. When it is fully grown, pull it up and eat it." In that simple cycle lies the essence of life. It is difficult to worry about inflation while carefully thinning out a row of carrot plants, impossible to be hurried while waiting for pears to ripen and not easy to turn over the soil and reveal a healthy crop of Idaho potatoes without experiencing a sense of real satisfaction. That is why avid gardeners tend as a breed to be relaxed, patient and optimistic. As Bertrand Russell once observed, "Every time I talk to a savant I feel quite sure that happiness is no longer a possibility. Yet when I talk with my gardener, I'm convinced of the opposite."

Other ideas for atavistic regression were suggested by a group of Japanese government officials, university professors, journalists and sociologists who set out to study the best ways for their countrymen to use their leisure time to help them cope with the stresses of their everyday working lives. They recommended a return to the traditional pastimes of bonsai (dwarf tree culture), ikebana (flower arranging) or even simply "listening to the sigh of the wind in the trees."

Whatever way is chosen we can find relief from stress by temporarily returning to a simpler way of life more closely attuned to our rustic origins. Then we experience the *vis medicatrix naturae,* the healing power of nature.

22

THE VALUE OF EXPERIENCE

We all tend to fear the unknown. A child can be frightened by its shadow, and African warriors have been known to flee in terror when they first hear a disembodied voice issuing from a transistor radio. Eventually familiarity with these everyday objects breeds a healthy contempt. We can, if we want to, overcome our natural inhibitions and learn to handle lions, charm snakes, climb steeples or walk on burning coals. To begin with we may experience fear, but with increasing practice we can perform these feats with less and less anxiety.

Ideally this confidence should be gained at an early age. Research workers set out to make infant rats neurotic by subjecting them to rough handling and mild electric shocks, but discovered that this early exposure to stress merely made them more courageous. It was the youngsters brought up in a protected, pampered environment who proved timid in later life and showed signs of exaggerated fear. Close parallels can be seen in the upbringing of human children. Analysis shows that many of the world's great leaders and men of daring were brought up in conditions of physical hardship or emotional deprivation which forced them to develop qualities of self-reliance at an early age. This is part of the rationale of the traditional British preparatory school which takes young boys from the protection of their mothers and offers them instead a toughening regime of harsh discipline, cold showers, drafty dormitories, early morning cross-country runs, boxing lessons and vigorous team sports. This echoes the training of the young men of Sparta, who were taken from their homes at the age of seven and subjected to a strict, state-run program of physical and military training. This made them, as adults, indifferent to danger and fear and models of toughness and spartan endurance. Similar principles are applied to the training of soldiers during their weeks of initial training. Here they are submitted to stringent discipline, fatigue, obstacle courses, forced marches and exhausting endurance tests. A man who has proved his ability to withstand these arduous tests has fewer qualms about his ability to survive the rigors of war. In the same way the businessman who has known adversity and been toughened in the hard school of personal experience develops an inner calm and assurance that book learning alone cannot provide. If he has survived on a shoestring he is less likely to feel threatened if he is temporarily out of work. If he has built his own business up from scratch, and had to peddle his own products from door to door, type his own letters and make his own coffee, he is less likely to be thrown into a spin later on when his ace salesman quits without giving adequate notice, his secretary falls sick and the office vending machine breaks down and fails to produce his early morning cup of coffee.

Ideally a gradual introduction should be made to tasks involving high levels of stress. Politicians should serve an apprenticeship in local politics and a succession of junior administrative posts before they are expected to tackle the enormous responsibility of a federal government appointment. In this way they learn to take the responsibility in their stride. Paratroopers, before they make their first descent from a plane, learn to fall in the gym and are then taken through a number of practice jumps from a tower. Tests show that, using this training schedule, anxiety lessens as experience grows. One psychologist asked trainee paratroopers to assess on a ten-point scale the amount of fear they experienced as they jumped from the thirty-foot training tower. On average the group reported a gradual decline of anxiety from six points on their first jump to three points on their seventh jump.

Even mock maneuvers help reduce anxiety. By the repeated practice of emergency drills we can become more confident of our ability to cope with a specific crisis. This explains the value of fire drills, boardroom games, mock examinations and the simulated accidents used to train first-aid workers. These school us for disaster and increase the probability that we will react calmly and effectively if an emergency occurs. The same applies to situations which provide a lesser threat.

The frustrations we meet in life have a positive value only if they sting us into taking purposeful, problem-solving action. This can only occur if we have the experience and technical skill to overcome the source of irritation. If you happen to be technically illiterate, and find the inside of a car as incomprehensible as Max Planck's original dissertation in German on the Quantum Theory, you are likely to suffer a degree of bewildered annoyance every time your car breaks down. If the engine stalls on the way to visit your in-laws, you may swear, beat the steering wheel in disgust or shout at your wife for wanting to make the trip in the first place, but you are unlikely to take the requisite action of lifting up the hood and correcting whatever has caused the fault. Only experience and the necessary technical skills enable us to cope effectively with frustrations in a crisis. If we accidentally fall out of a boat into deep water we are likely to experience a certain degree of stress. But the amount of anxiety we feel bears little relationship to our personality, upbringing, self-esteem or early childhood trauma. What really matters at the time is whether or not we can swim. So it is with life's other stresses and strains. Our ability to survive disappointments, deprivations and disasters depends to a large extent on our acquired social and technical skills.

A machine operator may be given hours of instruction on how to **handle** a complicated machine, while his boss receives no training at all to help him handle a staff of thousands. Whatever his natural aptitude for dealing with people, the chances are he can improve and extend his social skills. He may be expert at handling highly motivated technical staff but hopeless at coaxing a reasonable day's work from casual laborers. He may be a tough boardroom negotiator but at a complete loss when faced with an hysterical secretary. He may have a gift for staff selection, showing an uncanny knack for finding round pegs to fill round jobs, but lack the equally important ability of prying square pegs from round holes. Unless something is done to extend his skills he is likely to jog along, constantly repeating a few tried and tested behavioral routines which may have worked in the past but which are totally inappropriate for the task in hand. In this he is like a tired museum guide who automatically mumbles through his set spiel even when some of his party are deaf and the remainder non-English-speaking Arabs.

To reduce the stress of human interaction we need to

enhance our social fluency. Some find this can be done by undertaking a long course of personal analysis, by joining an encounter group, or by partaking in any of the many group exercises designed by industrial psychologists to foster what they frequently refer to as interactive skills. This fluency can also be obtained on the job, by spreading our circle of human encounters, and becoming more aware of ourselves and our interaction with others. The same applies to the acquisition of other managerial skills.

It is possible to learn the art of inventory control from a book, or consider the marketing of a revolutionary new product as a technical exercise or managerial game. But this is far less effective than learning on the job. This is the method favored by Reg Revans, the founder of the new management technique known as Action Learning. Revans, a seventy-year-old ex-Olympic hurdler, is critical of business schools and their preoccupation with theory and classroom studies. This formal training is no substitute for practical experience, he believes, and he advocates "using the real problems of the organization as learning opportunities." Industry's great need is for executives skilled at handling real-life problems with ease and equanimity. This can only come with practice. In a recent study the British Government–sponsored Training Services Agency listed a manager's three essential skills as being:

1. The technical expertise relevant to his job (marketing, engineering, production, accountancy, law).
2. The psychosocial skills of problem-solving, decision-making, communication and management.
3. The ability to go on learning.

The first prerequisite may be obtained through routine business studies, but the second and third can only be acquired through practical experience. One way of obtaining this breadth of practical knowledge, favored by Action Learning, is to send managers to solve problems in outside companies. Thus the marketing manager of a large poultry group was asked to see how an international telecommunications company could make the transfer of their staff from one country to another more acceptable, while a vice-president of an American subsidiary of the telecommunications firm was given the task of improving the poultry group's share of the market for chicken feed. The net result was that the organizations enjoyed a valuable, although sometimes slightly traumatic, scrutiny of their problems by a fresh, unprejudiced outside mind; while the men themselves gained experience, understanding and heightened self-confidence in their ability to cope with a variety of unusual dilemmas. Experience of this kind is never wasted. J. Paul Getty found his knowledge of constructing oil rigs invaluable when he had to turn his attention to building airplanes during the war; and when it was necessary to build a miniature city in the desert to house his employees in the Middle East oilfields he drew heavily on his earlier experience of hotel building and real estate.

Like a chess master, the executive needs to have experience of every possible strategy, end-game play and opening gambit. Then he can go into battle with the confidence that he is prepared for every eventuality, and can say, like the Russian chess master Elim Bogolybubou, "When I play white I win because I have the first move. When I play black I win because I am Bogolybubou."

These experiential skills can be developed by pursuing the following strategies:

- *Enter the lion's den.* Never dodge a crisis or shirk a difficult decision. You can never learn to swim unless you are prepared to get your feet wet. Confidence comes not from dilemmas evaded but from challenges overcome. In the past surgeons acquired their skills by going from battle to battle, doing their best to heal the wounded and picking up valuable expertise as they went. In the same way an executive can improve his trouble-shooting skills by keeping close to the battlefield. The legendary "Red" Adair, the world's foremost authority on controlling oil well fires and blow outs, gained his unrivaled knowledge over a period of forty years during which time he personally extinguished over a thousand fires. Experience of this nature inevitably gives a man confidence to cope during moments of crisis.

- *Follow a policy of a regular job rotation.* The ideal manager is a generalist with a wide scope of skills at his disposal. If the job you're in does not allow you to develop these managerial skills, change your job at regular intervals or opt for a smaller company where you are forced to be a jack-of-all-trades. Alternatively adopt a conscious policy of job rotation and role reversal. If you are in charge of product development try to spend some time on the road with one of the company's salesmen; if you are in public relations spend a day answering calls on the firm's switchboard. This is invaluable experience. And whenever possible use your leisure time to fill the cultural gaps. For instance, if you are in a position of authority by day join a choir or amateur drama group and see what it is like to be subjected to the discipline of a choir master or director. If you constantly find yourself at loggerheads with union officials, spend an occasional evening at a union meeting. Drink with their officials in the local bar afterward and try to see what makes them tick. Then, perhaps, you will experience less stress when next you meet them around the conference table.

- *Read all you can about human behavior.* Much of the stress of an executive's life comes from interpersonal conflicts. The more he learns about human behavior the greater his understanding and the less his confusion and stress. J. Paul Getty, in *How to Be a Successful Executive*, placed great emphasis on the value of a broad-based arts education for executives. Specialists can always be hired. The manager needs to have wide horizons and develop a deep insight and understanding of the structure and dynamics of society as a whole. Getty himself greatly benefited from the time he spent studying classics at Oxford University. "They helped me to be a better man—and a better businessman," he claimed. "My exposure to a wide variety of liberal arts subjects made my mind more flexible, more receptive to new ideas, more readily aware of changing circumstances and, at the same time, more convinced of what constitutes real and lasting values."

The Bell Telephone Company shares the same opinion. They grew concerned because so many of their talented and conscientous young men showed the "trained incapacity" of the narrow technical expert. They wanted to train managers who knew not only *how* to answer questions, but also *what* questions should be asked. So, in conjunction with the Institute of Humanistic Studies for Executives, they sent some of their key middle-managers on a ten-month liberal arts course with all expenses paid. At the end of the course they returned to their jobs and, according to one report, "They had more confidence and wanted greater responsibility. They could make better decisions because their attitude was more detached, critical, tolerant and objective; they could see all sides of a question and realized there was not always one solution. Although they had wider interests, they were still ambitious. In their private lives they became more interested in ideas and people, without becoming 'intellectuals.' They realized they owed something to themselves and their families as well as to the firm."

- *Study history.* An impressive number of the world's great leaders have been keen students of history. This has enabled them to see things in perspective and helped them learn from the wisdom of the past. It has also provided them with exemplars, men of outstanding courage, persistence and endeavor on whom they could model their lives.

- *Carry out an honest self-assessment* and rectify any deficiencies you find. If you suffer agonies every time you stand up to give an after-dinner speech, enroll in a class in public speaking. If your memory constantly plays you tricks take a course in pelmanism. If you're ill at ease in company read Dale Carnegie's book *How to Win Friends and Influence People*. Social skills such as these can be acquired.

By the time we are forty we are all a bundle of habits. Some of these habits are good and work for our advancement. Others are bad and hold us back and cause us needless anxiety and stress. Fortunately, none of these habits are fixed. We can modify our behavior if we choose. That is the message of this book. Stress is an integral and inescapable feature of human existence. Handle it wisely and it will enrich your life. Allow it to run amok and it will cause needless anxiety, sickness, fatigue and even premature death. The choice is yours.

BIBLIOGRAPHY

Ansoff, H. Igor, *Corporate Strategy*. (New York: McGraw-Hill, 1965)

Argyle, Michael, *The Psychology of Interpersonal Behavior*. (Harmondsworth, England: Penguin, 1970)

Argyle, Michael, *The Social Psychology of Work*. (Harmondsworth, England: Penguin, 1974)

Bennett, Arnold, *Mental Efficiency*. (Tadworth: World's Work, 1920)

Benson, Herbert, *The Relaxation Response*. (New York: William Morrow, 1975)

Brown, J.A.C., *The Social Psychology of Industry*. (Harmondsworth, England: Penguin, 1970)

Brown, Norman O., *Life Against Death*. (London: Routledge and Kegan Paul, 1959)

Carnegie, Dale, *How to Win Friends and Influence People*. (Tadworth: World's Work, 1953)

Carruthers, Malcolm, *The Western Way of Death*. (London: Davis-Poynter, 1974)

Dubos, René, *Man Adapting*. (New Haven: Yale University Press, 1966)

Duerr, Carl, *Management Kinetics*. (New York: McGraw-Hill, 1971)

Getty, J. Paul, *How to Be a Successful Executive*. (London: W. H. Allen, 1971)

Jacobson, E., *Progressive Relaxation*. (Chicago: University of Chicago, 1938)

Kearns, Joseph L., *Stress in Industry*. (Hove, England: Priory Press, 1973)

Knipe, Humphrey and Maclay, George, *The Dominant Man*. (London: Souvenir Press, 1973)

Levitt, Eugene E., *The Psychology of Anxiety*. (St. Albans, England: Staples Press, 1968)

Mackarness, Richard. *Not All in the Mind*. (London: Pan, 1976)

Maier, Norman R. F., *Psychology in Industry*. (London: George C. Harrap, 1947)

Maslow, Abraham, *The Farther Reaches of Human Nature*. (New York: Viking, 1971)

Morris, Desmond, *The Human Zoo*. (London: Jonathan Cape, 1969)

Norfolk, Donald, *The Habits of Health*. (New York: St. Martins Press, 1977)

Oates, Wayne E., *Confessions of a Workaholic*. (Mountain View: World, 1971)

Ogilvie, Sir Heneage, *The Tired Business Man*. (Springfield: Charles C. Thomas, 1964)

Page, Martin, *The Company Savage*. (London: Cassell, 1972)

Pahl, J.M. and R.E., *Managers and Their Wives*. (Hardmondsworth, England: Penguin, 1972)

Peter, Laurence J. and Hull, Raymond, *The Peter Principle*. (London: Souvenir Press, 1969)

Reich, Charles A., *The Greening of America*. (New York: Random House, 1970)

Sargant, William, *Battle for the Mind*. (London: William Heinemann, 1957)

Schindler, John A., *How to Live on 365 Days a Year*. (Englewood Cliffs, N.J.: Prentice Hall, 1954)

Schultz, J.H. and Luthe, W., *Autogenic Training*. (New York: Grune and Stratton, 1959)

Selye, Hans, *The Stress of Life*. (Burnt Mill, England: Longmans, 1957)

Selye, Hans, *Stress Without Distress*. (Philadelphia: J.B. Lippincott, 1974)

Storr, Anthony, *Human Aggression*. (Hardmondsworth, England: Penguin, 1971)

Storr, Anthony, *The Integrity of the Personality*. (London: William Heinemann, 1960)

Toffler, Alvin, *Future Shock*. (New York: Random House, 1970)

Whyte, William H., *The Organization Man*. (New York: Simon and Schuster, 1956)

Wright, H. Beric, *Executive Ease and Dis-ease*. (Epping, England: Gower Press, 1975)

Wyllie, I.G., *The Self-Made Man in America*. (London: Signet, 1964)

INDEX

INVENTORY 1983